高等医药院校教材

供基础、临床、预防、口腔医学类专业用

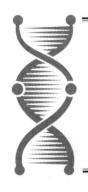

细胞生物学与医学遗传学实验教程

第3版

主　编　蔡绍京　姚瑞芹　夏米西努尔·伊力克
副主编　沈　滟　袁　芳　宋远见　贺　怡
编　委　（按姓氏笔画排序）

李　风	徐州医科大学
希林古丽·吾守尔	新疆医科大学
沈　滟	河南科技大学
宋远见	徐州医科大学
武秀香	徐州医科大学
姚瑞芹	徐州医科大学
贺　怡	新疆第二医学院
袁　芳	新疆医科大学
夏米西努尔·伊力克	新疆医科大学
高　蒙	河南科技大学
曹　青	河南科技大学
蔡绍京	徐州医科大学
熊　晔	徐州医科大学

人民卫生出版社

·北　京·

版权所有，侵权必究！

图书在版编目（CIP）数据

细胞生物学与医学遗传学实验教程 / 蔡绍京，姚瑞芹，夏米西努尔·伊力克主编 . —3 版 . —北京：人民卫生出版社，2021.8（2023.9 重印）

ISBN 978-7-117-31695-8

Ⅰ . ①细… Ⅱ . ①蔡…②姚…③夏… Ⅲ . ①细胞生物学 – 实验 – 医学院校 – 教材②医学遗传学 – 实验 – 医学院校 – 教材 Ⅳ . ①R329.2–33②R394–33

中国版本图书馆 CIP 数据核字（2021）第 149454 号

| 人卫智网 | www.ipmph.com | 医学教育、学术、考试、健康，购书智慧智能综合服务平台 |
| 人卫官网 | www.pmph.com | 人卫官方资讯发布平台 |

细胞生物学与医学遗传学实验教程
Xibao Shengwuxue yu Yixue Yichuanxue Shiyan Jiaocheng
第 3 版

主　　编：蔡绍京　姚瑞芹　夏米西努尔·伊力克
出版发行：人民卫生出版社（中继线 010-59780011）
地　　址：北京市朝阳区潘家园南里 19 号
邮　　编：100021
E - mail：pmph @ pmph.com
购书热线：010-59787592　010-59787584　010-65264830
印　　刷：天津画中画印刷有限公司
经　　销：新华书店
开　　本：787 × 1092　1/16　印张：8.5　插页：1
字　　数：212 千字
版　　次：2011 年 1 月第 1 版　2021 年 8 月第 3 版
印　　次：2023 年 9 月第 8 次印刷
标准书号：ISBN 978-7-117-31695-8
定　　价：28.00 元

打击盗版举报电话：010-59787491　E-mail：WQ @ pmph.com
质量问题联系电话：010-59787234　E-mail：zhiliang @ pmph.com

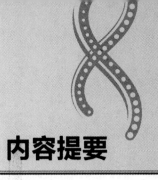

内容提要

　　《细胞生物学与医学遗传学实验教程》(第3版)由新疆医科大学、新疆第二医学院、河南科技大学和徐州医科大学专家教授共同编写。全书包括本科生细胞生物学实验、医学遗传学实验、留学生细胞生物学实验(英文)及附录的动物实验基本知识三部分。本实验教程的特点是介绍实验原理、实验目的和要求简明扼要,介绍实验操作过程详尽、明了;"实验操作"后的分析思考题及实验报告有助于学生加深对相关理论知识和实验内容的理解和掌握。

　　本实验教程包含细胞生物学实验和医学遗传学实验的经典内容,对大多数医学院校本科生的细胞生物学、医学遗传学及留学生的细胞生物学实验教学均具有广泛的适用性,也可供医学相关专业的研究生选用。

第3版前言

细胞生物学和医学遗传学是高等医学教育的重要基础课程,也是实验性很强的两门学科。通过实验教学,不仅能使学生掌握实验技能、加深对相关知识的理解和掌握,而且有助于培养学生实事求是的科学态度、严谨细致的工作作风以及分析问题和解决问题的能力。

《细胞生物学与医学遗传学实验教程》(第2版)于2014年7月出版,至今已近7年。为适应医学教育教学改革及留学生细胞生物学实验教学的需要,新疆医科大学、新疆第二医学院、河南科技大学和徐州医科大学的细胞生物学与医学遗传学教师对《细胞生物学与医学遗传学实验教程》(第2版)进行了修订。

本次修订依据4校本科生细胞生物学与医学遗传学实验教学及留学生细胞生物学实验教学的要求进行。全书分三部分,第一部分是本科生实验,共17个实验,能满足医学院校医学相关专业及生物科学、生物技术专业的细胞生物学、医学遗传学及遗传学的实验教学要求;第二部分是留学生实验,共8个实验,能满足留学生的细胞生物学实验教学需要;第三部分是附录的动物实验基本知识,除满足细胞生物学与医学遗传学实验需要外,也为基础医学各学科实验课所涉及的动物实验打下基础。

本实验教程的编写注重适应各参编院校实验课的开设需要。各参编院校实验课时差别较大,实验课的开设内容也不尽相同,有些实验是各校均开设的,有些实验仅个别院校开设。为满足各校实验课的需要,即使是个别院校的实验内容,我们也将其编入。需要说明的是,本书中的每个实验主要依据内容的相关性排定,并非代表一次实验课的内容。鉴于各校每次实验课的课时不同,实验总课时也不同,因此,各校可根据具体情况选取相应的实验内容教学。

本实验教程除能满足参编院校的实验教学需要外,对大多数医学院校本科生的细胞生物学、医学遗传学及留学生的细胞生物学教学均具有广泛的适用性。修订后的《细胞生物学与医学遗传学实验教程》(第3版)除增加留学生的细胞生物学实验内容外,本科生的实验内容也进行了优化,并删除了部分不常用的实验内容。

参加《细胞生物学与医学遗传学实验教程》(第3版)修订工作的各位编者,均长期工作在教学一线,具有丰富的教学经验。各位编者本着对学生负责的态度,对相关的实验内容及英文仔细推敲、精益求精、一丝不苟、数易其稿。尽管如此,由于医学科学的迅猛发展及编写人员的水平所限,书中难免有不足及疏漏之处,真诚期望同行专家及使用本实验教程的师生提出宝贵意见,以便再版时修正。

蔡绍京

2021年4月

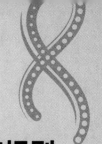

实验课要求与实验室规则

"细胞生物学"和"医学遗传学"是医学教育中两门重要的基础学科,也是实验性很强的学科;细胞生物学实验课和医学遗传学实验课是整个课程教学的重要组成部分。为保证实验的顺利进行,并获得预期的实验结果,特提出如下实验课要求及实验课规则。

一、实验课要求

1. 通过实验,验证和巩固相关的理论知识,加深对理论知识的理解。

2. 通过实验,培养实事求是、严谨细致的科学态度,科学的思维方法和独立思考、独立工作的能力。

3. 通过具体的实验操作,掌握两门实验课的基本实验方法和基本实验技能。

4. 每次实验课前,要认真预习实验教程及教材的相关内容,明确实验目的、要求,对实验内容、实验原理、实验方法和步骤,做到心中有数。

5. 实验过程中,要按照实验步骤,细心操作,仔细观察,做好实验记录,分析实验结果,培养自己分析问题和解决问题的能力,并认真完成实验报告。

二、实验室规则

1. 遵守纪律,不迟到、早退;实验中途如需外出,应向老师请假。

2. 进入实验室,要带齐学习用品(包括绘图用品),穿好白大衣,按指定座位入座。

3. 实验过程要保持肃静,不得在实验室内大声喧哗及随意走动,不做与实验无关的事。

4. 爱护仪器、标本和设备;如遇仪器故障或操作不灵,应及时报告老师,以便修理或更换,不要自行拆卸;各实验小组实验器材不得互相调换。

5. 注意节约实验材料、药品以及水、电资源,损坏仪器或标本应按规定赔偿。

6. 保持实验室内清洁;实验结束后,各实验小组必须认真清理各自的实验台面,将器材清洗并清点后整齐摆放;值日生负责清扫室内卫生,实验废弃物放置到指定地点,关好门窗、水电。

三、妥善保存本实验教程

本实验教程供"细胞生物学"和"医学遗传学"两门课程的实验教学使用,请在"细胞生物学"实验课程全部结束后,妥善保存本实验教程,后期的"医学遗传学"课程的实验课还要使用。

目录

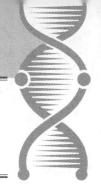

第一部分　本科生实验

实验1　普通光学显微镜

【目的要求】

1. 熟悉普通光学显微镜的主要构造及其性能。
2. 掌握低倍镜及高倍镜的使用方法。
3. 初步掌握油镜的使用方法。
4. 熟悉普通光学显微镜的维护方法。

【实验原理】

光学显微镜,简称光镜,是经光源照明,利用凸透镜的放大成像原理,使微小物体形成放大影像的设备。显微镜发明和使用已有400多年历史。1590年前后,荷兰的Janssen父子研制出了放大10倍的原始显微镜;1665年,英国物理学家R. Hooke研制出性能较好的显微镜并用它发现了细胞。400多年来,经过不断改进,显微镜的结构和性能逐步完善。目前常用的是双筒倾斜式显微镜,除少数应用反光镜采光外,大多数具有电光源。除了广泛使用的普通光学显微镜外,还有相差显微镜、暗视野显微镜、荧光显微镜和激光扫描共聚焦显微镜等具有特殊功能或用途的光镜。形形色色的光镜外形和结构差异较大,但其基本构造和工作原理是相似的。一台普通光学显微镜主要由机械系统和光学系统两部分构成,而作为显微镜核心部分的光学系统则主要包括目镜、物镜、聚光器和反光镜(或电光源)等部件(图1-1)。

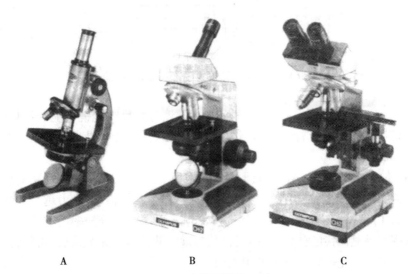

图1-1　光学显微镜示例

A. 单筒直立式;B. 单筒倾斜式;C. 双筒倾斜式。

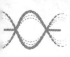

目镜和物镜的结构虽然比较复杂,但它们的作用都相当于一个凸透镜。由于被检标本是放在物镜下方1~2倍焦距之间,故物镜可使标本形成一个倒立的放大实像,该实像正好位于目镜的下焦点(焦平面)之内,故目镜可进一步将它放大成一个虚像,通过调焦可使虚像落在眼睛的明视距离处,从而在视网膜上形成一个直立的实像。光镜中被放大的倒立虚像与视网膜上直立的实像是相吻合的,该虚像看起来好像在离眼睛 25cm 处(图 1-2)。

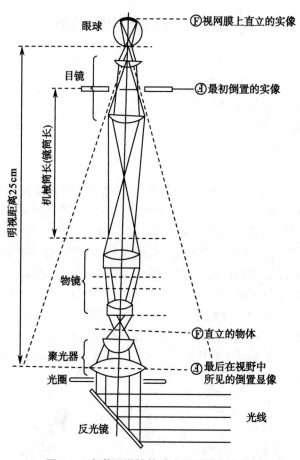

图 1-2 光学显微镜的放大原理及光路图

分辨率、放大率、数值孔径、焦点深度和视场宽度等是反映光镜性能和质量的指标。这些性能指标都有一定限度,彼此既相互作用又相互制约,改善或提高某方面的性能,往往会使另一性能降低。

分辨率(resolution,R)是光镜最重要的性能指标,是指在 25cm 的明视距离处,能区分开被检物体上两个质点间的最小距离。因此,分辨率越小,说明分辨能力越高。据测定,人眼的分辨率约为 100μm,而光镜的分辨率可达 0.2μm。显微镜的分辨率由物镜的分辨率决定,物镜的分辨率就是显微镜的分辨率,而目镜与显微镜的分辨率无关,它只将物镜已分辨的影像进行第二次放大。光镜的分辨率可用式(1-1)计算:

$$R=0.61\lambda/N.A.=0.61\lambda/n \cdot \sin(\alpha/2) \tag{1-1}$$

式(1-1)中 λ 为照明光源的波长,可见光的最短波长为 0.4μm。N.A. 代表数值孔径,数值等于物镜和被检样品之间介质的折射率(n)与镜口角(α)一半的正弦值的乘积,即

N.A.=n·sin(α/2)。n 的最大值为 1.5(香柏油为介质),镜口角是指位于物镜光轴上标本的一个点发出的光线延伸到物镜前透镜的有效直径的两端所形成的夹角,镜口角越大,进入物镜的光线越多,sin(α/2) 的最大值为 1(α=180°)。因此,N.A. 的最大值为 n·sin(α/2)=1.5 × 1=1.5。

由式(1-1)可知,物镜的 N.A. 决定一台显微镜的主要光学性能,N.A. 越大,分辨率就越小,显微镜的分辨能力就越强,显微镜的光学性能也越好。但 N.A. 与焦点深度(即当显微镜对标本的某一点或平面准焦时,焦点平面上下影像清晰的距离或范围)成反比,因此,并非 N.A. 越大越好。物镜的 N.A. 通常标刻在物镜的周缘。

使用低倍镜和高倍镜时,空气为介质,n 值为 1.0;使用油镜时,香柏油为介质,n 值为 1.5 (n 的最大值)。因此,油镜的 N.A. 大于低倍镜和高倍镜,即油镜的分辨能力高于低倍镜和高倍镜。目前,在实用范围内,物镜(油镜)的最大 N.A. 为 1.4。将 λ 和 N.A. 代入分辨率计算公式,可得 R=0.61 × 0.4μm/1.4 ≈ 0.174μm,即显微镜的最大分辨率约为 0.2μm。另外,由于空气与玻片的密度不同,当光线通过玻片与物镜镜头间的空气介质时,发生散射,降低了视野的照明度;而玻片和香柏油的折射率相近,当光线通过时,几乎不发生折射,增加了视野的进光量,故使用油镜观察标本时,物像会更加清晰。

放大率或放大倍数是光镜性能另一重要参数,光镜的总放大倍数等于目镜放大倍数与物镜放大倍数的乘积。

本次实验主要学习普通光学显微镜(以下简称显微镜)的基本结构、功能及使用方法。

【实验用品】

(一)材料

人血涂片或蟾蜍血涂片、蟾蜍脊髓横切面切片、羊毛(毛线)交叉装片、英文字母装片等。

(二)器材

显微镜、香柏油(或液体石蜡)、无水乙醇(或乙醚乙醇混合液)、擦镜纸。

【实验步骤】

一、熟悉显微镜的基本结构与功能

(一)机械系统

1. 镜筒　镜筒是安装在显微镜最上方的圆筒状结构,其上端装有目镜,下端与物镜转换器相连(图 1-3)。

2. 物镜转换器　物镜转换器又称旋转盘,是安装在镜筒下方的圆盘状结构,可顺时针及逆时针方向旋转,其上均匀分布有 3~4 个圆孔,可安装不同放大倍数物镜。转动物镜转换器可使不同的物镜到达工作位置(即与光路合轴)。

3. 镜臂　镜臂是支持镜筒和镜台的结构,下端与镜座相连,是取用显微镜时握持的部位。

4. 调焦器　调焦器也称调焦螺旋,是调节焦距的装置,位于镜臂的下方,分为粗调焦螺旋(大螺旋)和细调焦螺旋(小螺旋)两种。粗调焦螺旋可使载物台以较快速度或较大幅度升降,能迅速调节好焦距,使物像呈现在视野中,适用于低倍镜观察时的调焦。细调焦螺旋使载物台缓慢升降,升降的幅度不易被肉眼观察到,适用于高倍镜和油镜的焦距精细调节,也适用于观察同一标本的不同焦平面。

5. 载物台　载物台也称镜台,是位于物镜转换器下方的方形平台,用于放置被观察的

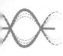

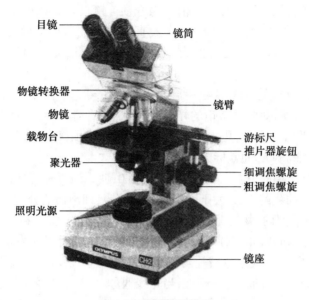

图 1-3　显微镜结构图

玻片标本。载物台的中央有圆形的通光孔,来自下方的光线经此孔照射到标本上。在载物台上装有标本移动器,也称推片器,其上安装的弹簧夹用于固定玻片标本,旋动推片器的两个旋钮,可使玻片标本前后或左右移动。

在推片器上附有纵、横游标尺,用以标记标本的位置。游标尺由主标尺(A)和副标尺(B)组成,副标尺的分度为主标尺的 9/10。使用时,先看副标尺的 0 点位置,再看主、副标尺刻度线的重合点,依据重合点即可读出准确的数值。图 1-4 中所示的数值应为 26.4。

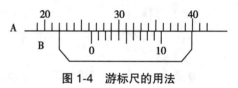

图 1-4　游标尺的用法

6. 镜座　镜座位于最底部,是整台显微镜的基座,用于支持和稳定镜体。

(二)光学系统

光学系统包括目镜、物镜、聚光器、反光镜(或电光源)等。

1. 目镜　目镜又称接目镜,安装在镜筒的上端,能将物镜所放大的物像进一步放大。每台显微镜通常配置 3~4 个不同放大倍数的目镜,如"×5""×10"和"×15"(数字表示放大倍数)目镜,可根据不同需要选择使用,最常用的是"×10"目镜。为方便指示视野中的某一结构,可将一小段细金属丝黏附在目镜内视场光阑上作为指针;另外,还可在视场光阑上安装目镜测微尺。

2. 物镜　物镜也称接物镜,安装在物镜转换器上。每台显微镜一般有 3~4 个不同放大倍数的物镜,物镜是显微镜最主要的光学部件,决定显微镜分辨率的大小。常用物镜的放大倍数有"×4""×10""×40"(或"×45")和"×100"等几种。一般将"×4""×10"物镜称为低倍镜,将"×40"或"×45"物镜称为高倍镜,将"×100"物镜称为油镜(这种镜头在使用时其顶端需浸在香柏油或液体石蜡中)。在每个物镜的周缘通常都标有能反映其主要性能的参数(图 1-5),主要有放大倍数和数值孔径(如 10/0.25、40/0.65 和 100/1.25)、该物镜所要求的镜筒长度和盖玻片厚度(160/0.17,单位为 mm);另外,在油镜上还常标有"油"或"oil"字样。

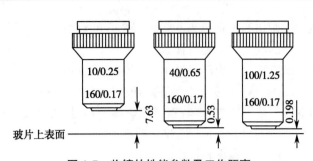

图1-5 物镜的性能参数及工作距离

注:两箭头间距离为工作距离,单位为mm。

不同物镜有不同的工作距离,所谓工作距离是指显微镜处于工作状态(焦距调好、物像清晰)时,物镜最下端与盖玻片上表面之间的距离(图1-5)。物镜的放大倍数与其工作距离成反比。当低倍镜调节到工作距离后,可直接转换成高倍镜或油镜,然后只需旋动细调焦螺旋,便可见到清晰的物像。不同放大倍数的物镜可从外形上区分,一般来说,低倍镜镜头最短,油镜镜头最长,而高倍镜的镜头长度介于两者之间。

3. 聚光器 聚光器位于载物台通光孔的下方,其主要功能是将光线集中到所要观察的标本上。聚光器由2~3个透镜组合而成,其作用相当于一个凸透镜,可将光线汇集成束。聚光器左下方通常有一调节旋钮,又称为聚光器孔径光阑调节手柄,用以升降聚光器;升高聚光器可使光线增强,反之则光线变弱。

4. 光圈 光圈位于聚光器下面,由一组金属薄片组合排列而成,拨动其外侧的小柄,可使光圈的孔径开大或缩小,以调节光线的强弱。有的显微镜光圈下方有滤光片框,可放置不同颜色的滤光片。

5. 反光镜 反光镜位于聚光器的下方,可向各方向转动,能将来自不同方向的光线反射到聚光器中。反光镜有平、凹两面:凹面镜有聚光作用,适于弱光和散射光下使用;光线较强时则选用平面镜。电光源显微镜,则使用调光螺旋调节光亮度。

二、学习显微镜的使用方法

(一) 低倍镜

1. 准备 将显微镜平稳地放置在自己座位正前方实验台上,镜座后缘离实验台边缘3~6cm。注意轻拿轻放。调节转凳的高度,至双眼能舒适地观察目镜。

2. 调光 先转动粗调焦螺旋,使载物台稍下降;再转动物镜转换器,使低倍镜转动到位(即低倍镜头对准通光孔);当镜头完全到位时,可听到轻微的顿挫声。开大光圈,上升聚光器到适当位置(以聚光器上方透镜平面稍低于载物台平面的高度为宜),将反光镜凹面转向光源;然后,双眼注视目镜,同时调节反光镜的角度,使视野内的光线均匀、亮度适中。如果使用电光源显微镜,则使用调光螺旋调节光亮度。

3. 置片 取需要观察的玻片标本,先对着光线用肉眼观察,了解标本的全貌;然后将玻片有盖玻片的一面朝上,放置到载物台上,用推片器上的弹簧夹固定好;最后,旋动推片器螺旋,使需要观察的标本部位处于通光孔中央。

4. 调焦 用眼睛从侧面注视低倍镜头与玻片的距离,同时调节粗调焦螺旋使载物台上升,直至低倍镜头距玻片标本的距离约0.5cm;然后,双眼自目镜观察,同时慢慢转动粗调焦螺旋使载物台下降直至视野中出现物像为止;最后,转动细调焦螺旋,使视野中的物像清晰。

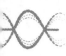

此种状态称为准焦状态,调焦的过程称为准焦。每个人的双眼瞳距不同,可通过调节两目镜轴间的距离,使视场重合形成完整的圆形视场。

调焦时,如果镜头与玻片的距离已超过 1cm 还未见到物像,应查找原因,加以纠正:①若物镜未完全转动到位,镜头未对准通光孔,应将物镜转动到位后再观察;②若标本在视野外,应移动推片器,使标本移至视野中央;③若粗调焦螺旋转动过快,越过了焦点,应缓缓回旋粗调焦螺旋;④若视野内光线过强,标本染色浅或标本未染色,应将光线适当调暗。不管是何种原因,都应严格按上述调焦步骤重新操作。

(二)高倍镜

1. 选择目标　在使用高倍镜前,应先用低倍镜寻找到需进一步观察的物像,并将其移至视野中央。

2. 换用高倍镜　为防止镜头碰撞玻片,转动物镜转换器时,要从显微镜的侧面注视,缓慢地将高倍镜转动到位,即高倍镜头对准通光孔。

3. 调焦　高倍镜转动到位后,视野中一般可见到不太清晰的物像。此时,只需稍稍调节细调焦螺旋,便可使物像清晰。若视野内亮度不够,可上升聚光器、开大光圈及调节反光镜的角度(电光源显微镜可增加光亮度)。

如果换用高倍镜时,镜头碰到玻片,此时不可强行转动,应查找原因并加以纠正。常见原因包括:①玻片放反;②玻片过厚;③高倍镜头松动;④低倍镜未准焦等。如果排除这些因素后,高倍镜头仍触碰到玻片,则为高倍镜头过长,可能为非原装高倍镜。此时应先将载物台下降,再换用高倍镜头,然后,在眼睛的注视下,将载物台升高至高倍镜头接近盖玻片;最后,在观察目镜的同时用粗调焦螺旋缓慢地使载物台下降;看到物像后,再用细调焦螺旋准焦。

由于制造工艺上的原因,许多显微镜的低倍镜视野中心与高倍镜视野中心往往存在一定的偏差。因此,在从低倍镜转换到高倍镜观察标本时,常会给观察者迅速找到标本造成一定困难。可通过绘制偏心图的方法解决这个问题。具体做法是:在高倍镜下找到羊毛交叉点并将其移至视野中央,换低倍镜观察羊毛交叉点所在视野的位置,该位置就是偏心位置。反复操作几次,找出准确的偏心位置并绘出偏心图。在使用该台显微镜的高倍镜观察标本前,应在低倍镜下将需进一步放大的物像移至偏心位置,再转换高倍镜观察,这样,所需观察的目标就正好处在视野中央了。

(三)油镜

1. 选择目标　将低倍镜或高倍镜下观察到的、并需要进一步放大的物像移至视野中央。

2. 调光　将聚光器上升至较高位置并将光圈开至最大(油镜所需光线较强)。

3. 换用油镜　转动物镜转换器,移开低倍镜或高倍镜,在玻片标本正对通光孔的部位滴一滴香柏油(或液体石蜡),然后在眼睛的注视下,将油镜转动到位,此时油镜的下端应正好浸在油滴中或与油滴接触。有的显微镜的油镜头过长,油镜头不能转动到位,此时,可先稍稍下降载物台,再将油镜头转到位,使油镜头下端浸入油滴中。

4. 调焦　双眼观察目镜的同时,小心而缓慢地转动细调焦螺旋使载物台下降,直至视野中出现清晰的物像。操作时不要反方向转动细调焦螺旋,以免镜头压碎标本或损坏镜头。在使用油镜观察过程中,如需更换观察目标,为防止高倍镜头沾油,可在低倍镜观察某一目标后直接换用油镜。

5. 擦拭　油镜使用结束后,必须及时将镜头上的油(或液体石蜡)擦拭干净。擦拭油镜头前,应将其转离通光孔,先用擦镜纸蘸少许无水乙醇(或乙醚乙醇混合液)擦 2 次,再用干净的擦镜纸擦 1 次。玻片上的油(或乙醚乙醇混合液)也需处理干净,如果是有盖玻片的永久制片,可直接用上述擦油镜头的方法擦净;如果是无盖玻片的标本,则用拉纸法除去载玻片上的油(或乙醚乙醇混合液),即先把一小片擦镜纸盖在含油(或乙醚乙醇混合液)玻片表面,再向擦镜纸上滴几滴无水乙醇,趁湿将擦镜纸向一侧拉,如此反复几次,即可将玻片上的油除去。

(四)注意事项

1. 取用显微镜时,应轻拿轻放。一手紧握镜臂,另一手托住镜座;禁用单手提拿,以避免零部件滑落。

2. 显微镜不可放置在实验台的边缘,应使镜座后缘离实验台边缘 3~6cm。课间离开座位时,应将显微镜的倾斜关节复原,镜头转离通光孔。

3. 不可随意拆卸显微镜上的零部件,以免丢失或损坏;目镜也不要随便取出,以防灰尘落入镜筒。

4. 要经常保持显微镜的清洁,显微镜的光学部分只能用擦镜纸轻轻擦拭,不可用纱布、手帕、普通纸张或手指擦拭,以避免磨损镜面。

5. 使用高倍镜和油镜观察时,只能调节细调焦螺旋,若转动粗调焦螺旋上升载物台,易导致镜头与玻片相撞,损坏镜头或玻片标本。需更换标本片时,应先转动粗调焦螺旋下降载物台,使镜头与载物台间距离拉开,然后再取下标本片。

6. 如需同老师或同学讨论视野中的某一结构,可用推片器将该结构移至指针尖端处;如果镜中未装指针,可将视野看成一个周缘带有刻度的钟面(如 3 点、6 点、9 点、12 点等),说明该结构位于钟面的几点钟位置。

7. 显微镜使用结束后应及时复原:先下降载物台,取下标本片,物镜转离通光孔;然后,上升载物台,使物镜与载物台相接近;使反光镜处于垂直位(或关闭电源),下降聚光器,关闭光圈。最后,将显微镜送还显微镜室。

三、操作练习

(一)观察英文字母装片、羊毛(毛线)交叉装片或其他标本片

观察字母装片时,先肉眼直接观察字母的方位和大小,然后放到低倍镜下观察。视野中字母的方位发生了什么变化? 标本移动的方向与视野中物像移动的方向有何不同?

观察羊毛交叉装片时,先在低倍镜下仔细观察两根羊毛的交叉点,然后将交叉点移至视野中央,换用高倍镜观察;利用细调焦螺旋分别对两根羊毛进行准焦,分辨出两根羊毛的上下位置。如果低倍视野中心与高倍视野中心存在偏差,可按前文介绍绘制偏心图的方法解决。

(二)观察人血涂片或蟾蜍血涂片

人血涂片上的血膜经瑞氏染液染色后呈蓝紫色,将蓝紫色的血膜对着通光孔,低倍镜下可看到大量密集的红细胞及少量散在的白细胞、血小板。换用高倍镜或油镜仔细观察:红细胞无核、中央色淡;白细胞均有核,核形态不一;血小板较小,形态不规则(图 1-6)。

(三)观察蟾蜍脊髓横切面切片

镜下可见脊髓前角运动神经细胞形态不规则,多呈三角形或星形;胞质染成蓝紫色,中央有圆形的细胞核,部分核内可看到大而圆的核仁;胞体向周围伸出的突起是树突。染色较深的小细胞是神经胶质细胞。

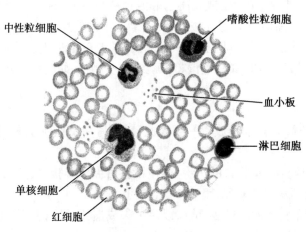

图 1-6 人血细胞

【分析思考】

1. 使用显微镜观察标本时,为什么必须按从低倍镜到高倍镜再到油镜的顺序进行?

2. 为什么低倍镜调焦前要先将低倍镜与标本表面的距离调节到 0.5cm?而油镜调焦前则先使油镜贴近标本表面?

3. 如果标本片放反了,可用高倍镜或油镜找到物像吗?

4. 低倍镜下见到的结构,换用高倍镜后找不到,怎么办?

5. 怎样才能准确而迅速地在高倍镜或油镜下找到目标?

6. 如果细调焦螺旋已转动至极限而物像仍不清晰,应该怎么办?

7. 如何判断视野中所见污点的来源?目镜对显微镜成像起什么作用?

【实验报告】

填图:标注图 1-7 中显微镜的部件名称。

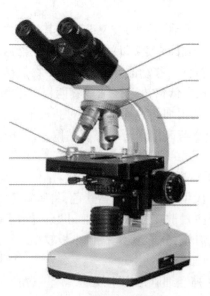

图 1-7 显微镜的部件

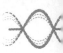

实验2 细胞的基本形态与结构

【目的要求】

1. 学习蟾蜍的处死方法。
2. 掌握临时装片的制片技术。
3. 熟悉光镜下动、植物细胞的基本形态和结构。
4. 初步掌握生物学绘图的方法。
5. 熟悉常用解剖器械的使用。

【实验原理】

1. 临时装片是将从生物体撕取或挑取的材料，现场制成的用于显微镜观察的标本片。临时装片的材料是从生物体获取的活的组织或细胞，经染色后即可用显微镜观察。根据材料的来源、结构不同，临时装片包括铺片、涂片及压片等。临时装片的制备简便易行，常用于观察细胞形态及基本结构。

2. 细胞的形态、结构与其功能密切相关，尤其是分化程度高的细胞。例如：具有收缩功能的肌细胞为细长形，具有感受刺激和传导冲动功能的神经细胞有长短不一的树枝状突起，哺乳类动物的红细胞为双凹圆盘形。尽管不同类型的细胞形态各异，但光镜下大多数细胞均包括质膜、细胞质和细胞核三部分结构；少数特化的细胞例外，如哺乳动物的红细胞成熟后细胞核消失。

【实验用品】

（一）材料

洋葱、蟾蜍、人口腔黏膜上皮细胞。

（二）器材

显微镜、载玻片、盖玻片、擦镜纸、清洁纱布、吸水纸、消毒牙签、解剖针、镊子、剪刀、眼科剪刀、培养皿、吸管。

（三）试剂

0.2%亚甲蓝、1%甲苯胺蓝、1%碘液、0.65%Ringer液（两栖类用）、瑞氏染液、生理盐水、蒸馏水。

【实验步骤】

（一）人口腔黏膜上皮细胞

1. 制片　在清洁的载玻片一端滴1滴0.2%亚甲蓝染液（或1%碘液），另一端滴1滴生理盐水，然后用消毒牙签的钝端轻轻刮取颊部内侧的口腔黏膜，将含有上皮细胞的牙签，平行放在载玻片上的染液中，来回滚动数次，使细胞落入染液中，染色2~3min；另取一牙签，以同样方法，使口腔上皮细胞落入生理盐水中。玻片两端均加盖玻片，盖玻片周围如有多余染液，可用吸水纸吸去。

2. 镜检　观察染色一端标本时，先用低倍镜寻找细胞，可见口腔黏膜上皮细胞染成蓝色（碘液染色为黄褐色）成群或散在分布。选择分散良好的细胞，换用高倍镜观察，可见细胞呈扁椭圆形、多边形或不规则形；卵圆形细胞核位于中央，染成深蓝色（或深黄褐色），部分细胞核中可见着色深的核仁；细胞质均匀一致，染成浅蓝色（或浅黄色），精细调焦后可见大小不等的颗粒（图2-1）。

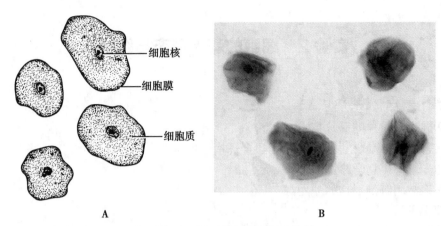

图 2-1　人口腔黏膜上皮细胞

A. 模式图；B. 显微结构图。

　　观察玻片另一端未染色的标本,并与染色的标本相比,镜下所见有何不同? 观察未染色标本时,如何调节视野的亮度,才能取得好的观察效果?

（二）洋葱表皮细胞

　　1. 制片　取一擦净的载玻片,滴 1 滴 1% 碘液；将洋葱鳞茎先剪成小块,然后取 1 块肉质鳞叶,剪成 3~4mm^2 的小块,再用镊子将其内表面表皮轻轻撕下,置于载玻片的染液中铺平；染色 2~3min 后,盖上盖玻片,用吸水纸吸去盖玻片周围多余的染液。

　　2. 镜检　低倍镜下,可见许多排列整齐、彼此相连的长菱形细胞。细胞表面有较厚的细胞壁,这是植物细胞的主要特征,细胞质膜因紧贴细胞壁而无法分辨。高倍镜下,可见细胞核呈椭圆形,多位于细胞中央,染成黄色；而成熟细胞的细胞核由于液泡的挤压,常位于细胞边缘；转动细调焦螺旋,可见核内有 1~2 个折光较强、染成深黄色的核仁。细胞质中可见 1 个或数个液泡及微细颗粒(图 2-2)。

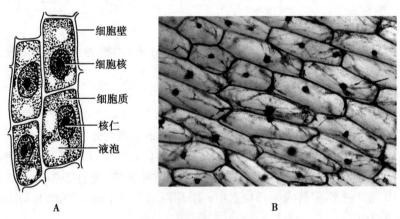

图 2-2　洋葱鳞茎表皮细胞

A. 模式图；B. 显微结构图。

（三）蟾蜍脊髓前角运动神经细胞

　　1. 制备压片　取蟾蜍 1 只,采用捣毁脊髓法处死(见附录),在口裂处剪去头部,除去延髓；将剪刀插入椎管暴露处,沿脊椎背面两侧分别纵向剪开椎管,暴露乳白色的脊髓。先用手术剪剪取长约 0.5cm 的中段脊髓,放在培养皿内,用两栖类 Ringer 液洗去血液并用吸水纸将液体吸净;然后将洗净的脊髓横断面朝上放在载玻片上,滴 1 滴 1% 甲苯胺蓝染液于标本上,染色 3~5min;最后盖上盖玻片,以拇指的腹面垂直向下用力按压标本,用吸水纸吸去溢出的染液,继续染色 5~10min。

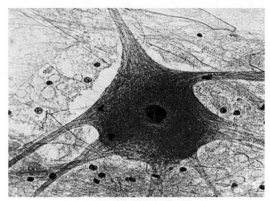

图 2-3　脊髓前角运动神经细胞

2. 镜检　镜下可见脊髓前角运动神经细胞的胞体很大,形态不规则,多呈三角形或星形;细胞质染成蓝紫色,中央有圆形的细胞核,部分细胞核内可见大而圆的核仁;胞体向周围伸出的多个细长突起是树突。脊髓前角运动神经细胞周围染色较深的小细胞是神经胶质细胞(图 2-3)。

(四)蟾蜍肝细胞

1. 制备压片　剪开蟾蜍胸腹腔,暴露出暗红色的肝脏,在肝脏的边缘处剪取一 2mm³ 左右组织块,放在培养皿内(注意:组织块一定不能太大)。用两栖类 Ringer 液清洗,并用镊子轻压将肝组织中的血挤出,然后放在载玻片上,用眼科剪刀将肝组织块进一步剪碎,弃去较大块组织,滴 1 滴 0.2% 亚甲蓝染液染色 3~5min,盖上盖玻片,用解剖针柄轻轻敲击盖玻片,继续染色 5~10min。

2. 镜检　镜下观察,可见肝细胞紧密排列,寻找单个的肝细胞或不重叠的肝细胞,可见肝细胞呈多边形,细胞核染成蓝色,注意核的形状和数目。

(五)蟾蜍血细胞

1. 制备血涂片　将蟾蜍心脏剪开一小口,用吸管吸取血液,滴 1 小滴于载玻片的右端,将另一张载玻片的一端放在血滴的左侧,然后右移至接触血滴,并使血滴沿其边缘展开,最后以 30°~45° 的角度平稳地将载玻片推向玻片的左端。推片时,推片的载玻片要与下方的载玻片贴紧,动作稍快,室温下晾干(图 2-4)。

2. 染色　取晾干的血涂片,在血膜薄而均匀的区域用蜡笔画一圆圈,在圆圈内滴加几滴瑞氏染液。约 1min 后,滴加等量的蒸馏水稀释染液,继续染 2~3min。自来水冲去染液,晾干后即可镜检。

3. 镜检　低倍镜下可见大量红细胞,少数白细胞。高倍镜下,红细胞为椭圆形,有核;白细胞核为圆形,紫蓝色(图 2-5)。

【分析思考】

1. 试说明蟾蜍脊髓前角运动神经细胞和肝细胞的形态结构特点,并比较二者的异同。

2. 试说明人红细胞和蟾蜍红细胞在形态结构上的异同点。

【实验报告】

1. 绘高倍镜下人口腔黏膜上皮细胞结构图。

2. 绘高倍镜下洋葱细胞形态结构图。

3. 绘高倍镜下蟾蜍脊髓前角运动神经细胞形态结构图。

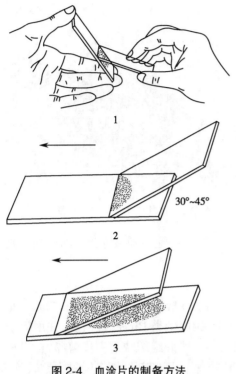

图 2-4　血涂片的制备方法

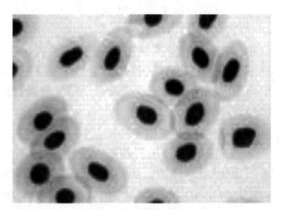

图 2-5　蟾蜍血细胞

【附】细胞生物学绘图方法及基本要求

细胞生物学绘图就是将光学显微镜下观察到的细胞结构真实地描绘下来。绘图方法及要求如下：

1. 布局合理,大小适中。考虑到图下方要标注图的名称、放大倍数,图的右侧要标出结构名称,因此,绘图区(即图的位置)应略偏上、略偏左。

2. 绘图务必真实、准确。绘图前应认真、仔细观察,所绘结构力求典型、清晰,要正确反映各部分结构的形态及毗邻关系。

3. 绘图时,先用软铅笔(HB 铅笔)轻轻绘出结构轮廓,修改确定后再用硬铅笔以粗细均匀的线条绘出全图;线条要连续、均匀,不能重复;细胞结构用大小均匀、疏密不同的圆点表示,不要涂暗影及其他美术处理。

4. 图的下方标注图的名称、放大倍数。从图中各主要结构处向右引出平行线,在平行线的末端标出结构名称;若不便引出平行线,可先引出斜线,再在斜线的末端引出平行线;斜引线间不能交叉,各平行线的末端要对齐。

5. 图中所标注的所有文字均要求用铅笔正楷书写,清晰、工整。

实验 3　细 胞 化 学

细胞化学(cytochemistry)是在保持细胞原有形态结构的基础上,利用化学试剂与细胞内的物质进行化学反应,在细胞局部形成有色沉淀物,显示细胞内生物大分子(如核酸、蛋白质、酶等),并通过显微镜观察,对细胞内生物大分子进行定性、定位、定量研究的细胞生物学实验研究技术。细胞化学是研究细胞成分的常用方法之一。

一、核酸的细胞化学

【目的要求】

1. 了解 Brachet 反应的原理。
2. 掌握细胞中 DNA 和 RNA 细胞化学染色方法。

【实验原理】

甲基绿(methyl green,MG)、派洛宁(pyronin,P)为带正电荷的碱性染料,可与带负电荷的核酸分子结合而显色。1940 年,布拉谢(Brachet)揭示了 MG-P 染色的组织化学原理,故此染色法也称为 Brachet 反应。

甲基绿和派洛宁的作用具有选择性。甲基绿带两个正电荷,对聚合程度高的双链 DNA 有强的亲和力,并且与 DNA 分子双螺旋结构上带负电荷的基团距离一致而易于结合,故甲基绿可使分布在细胞核中的 DNA 染成蓝色或绿色;派洛宁分子只带有一个正电荷,仅能和聚合程度低的单链 RNA 分子结合,使分布于胞质和核仁中的 RNA 染成红色。

这说明甲基绿和派洛宁对核酸的显色反应不是化学作用,而是与 DNA 和 RNA 的聚合程度有关,DNA 解聚到一定程度时也可与派洛宁结合而呈红色。细胞经甲基绿 - 派洛宁混合液处理后,其中的 DNA 和 RNA 呈现不同的显色反应,故可对细胞中的 DNA、RNA 进行定性、定位和定量分析。

【实验用品】

(一)材料

蟾蜍。

(二)器材

解剖器械、显微镜、载玻片、吸水纸、蜡笔、盖玻片。

(三)试剂

甲基绿 - 派洛宁染液、丙酮、丙酮与二甲苯(1:2)混合液、70% 乙醇、二甲苯、蒸馏水。

【实验步骤】

1. 取材与制片　蟾蜍血涂片的制备参见实验二。
2. 固定　将 1 张血涂片放入 70% 乙醇中固定 5~10min,取出后晾干。
3. 染色　用蜡笔在血涂片上血膜两端画线,框出染色部位。在血涂片表面滴加数滴甲基绿 - 派洛宁染液,染色 30min(注意:染液宜稍微多加些,染色过程中不能由于染液挥发致血涂片表面暴露)。
4. 冲洗　弃去血涂片上染液,用蒸馏水冲洗 2~3 次,用吸水纸吸干载玻片背面水分,但正面血膜处不要吸得过干。
5. 分色与透明　将血涂片依次放入纯丙酮中分色 2~3s(最多不可超过 10s,否则颜色褪去),丙酮、二甲苯混合液(1:2)中 5s,二甲苯中透明 5min。
6. 镜检　在低倍镜、高倍镜下找到物像后,换用油镜观察,可见细胞质染成红色,细胞核染成蓝绿色,而其中核仁染成红色。

【分析思考】

1. 简述 Brachet 反应显示 DNA 和 RNA 的原理。
2. 为什么蟾蜍红细胞的细胞质和细胞核可被甲基绿 - 派洛宁染液染成不同颜色?
3. 在 Brachet 反应中,细胞核和细胞质各被染上什么颜色? 如果能看到核仁,核仁应被染成什么颜色? 这种染色差异说明什么?

4. 细胞内 DNA 和 RNA 分别分布在细胞的哪些部位?

【实验报告】

1. 画出 Brachet 反应的蟾蜍红细胞图,分别标明细胞质、细胞核的颜色;根据自己的实验结果,解释处理片和未处理片中细胞核、细胞质的颜色差异。

2. 绘图表示蟾蜍红细胞中 DNA 和 RNA 的分布。

二、蛋白质的细胞化学

【目的要求】

1. 了解蛋白质的细胞化学反应原理。

2. 掌握细胞中酸性蛋白和碱性蛋白的细胞化学染色方法。

【实验原理】

1. 由于不同蛋白质分子中所带有的碱性基团(氨基)和酸性基团(羧基)的数量不同,因此,在不同的 pH 溶液中,整个蛋白质所带正电荷或负电荷就不同。在生理条件下,整个蛋白质带负电的为酸性蛋白质,带正电荷的为碱性蛋白质。因此,将标本经三氯醋酸处理提取核酸后,用不同 pH 的固绿染色,可使细胞内酸性和碱性蛋白质分别显示出来。

2. 细胞骨架是真核细胞中由蛋白质纤维构成的网络结构,由微丝、微管和中间丝构成,对细胞形态的维持,细胞的生长、运动、分裂、分化和物质运输等起重要作用。光学显微镜下观察细胞骨架结构的方法是先用非离子去垢剂 TritonX-100(聚乙二醇辛基苯醚)处理细胞,溶解细胞质膜、细胞壁、细胞内 95% 的可溶性蛋白质及全部脂质,但细胞骨架的蛋白质不被溶解和破坏而得到保存;再经固定和非特异性蛋白质染料考马斯亮蓝 R250 染色,则可在光镜下观察到清晰的细胞骨架结构。

在该实验条件下,微管结构不稳定,而直径 10nm 左右的中间丝太细,光镜下也无法分辨。因此,光镜下见到的细胞骨架实际上是多根微丝形成的微丝束,也称为应力纤维。

【实验用品】

(一) 材料

蟾蜍、洋葱鳞茎、人口腔黏膜上皮细胞。

(二) 器材

恒温水浴箱、离心机、电炉、显微镜、解剖器械、小烧杯、载玻片、盖玻片、吸水纸、染色缸、蜡笔、培养皿、吸管、牙签。

(三) 试剂

5% 三氯醋酸、10% 甲醛、0.1% 酸性固绿染液(pH 2.0)、0.1% 碱性固绿染液(pH 8.0)、6mmol/L PBS(pH 6.5)、磷酸氢二钠 - 柠檬酸缓冲液(pH 2.2)、磷酸盐缓冲液(pH 7.2)、磷酸氢二钠 - 柠檬酸缓冲液(pH 8.0)、M- 缓冲液(pH 7.2)、1% TritonX-100、0.2% 考马斯亮蓝 R250 染液、3% 戊二醛、70% 乙醇、生理盐水、蒸馏水。

【实验步骤】

(一) 酸性蛋白和碱性蛋白

1. 动物细胞

(1) 取材、制片:蟾蜍血涂片的制备参见实验二(或取已制备的蟾蜍血涂片 2 张)。

(2) 固定:将涂片放在 70% 乙醇中固定 5min,室温晾干。

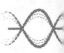

（3）三氯醋酸处理:将涂片放入 60℃ 5% 三氯醋酸中处理 30min,抽提去除核酸。取出涂片用自来水冲洗 3min 以上,直至标本上无三氯醋酸痕迹。注意:三氯醋酸残留会干扰固绿的染色,影响观察结果。

（4）染色:用吸水纸吸干玻片上水分,用蜡笔框出染色部位。拟显示酸性蛋白的涂片用 0.1% 酸性固绿染液（pH 2.0）染色 5~10min。拟显示碱性蛋白的涂片用 0.1% 碱性固绿染液（pH 8.0）染色 30~60min。这两张玻片染色后均经自来水冲洗,室温晾干。

（5）镜检:在低倍镜下找到物像后,换用高倍镜观察。高倍镜下可见,经酸性固绿染液染色的标本,细胞质和核仁被染成绿色,此即酸性蛋白质在细胞内的分布;经碱性固绿染液染色的标本,只有细胞核被染成绿色,此即核内参与染色体构成的组蛋白——碱性蛋白质在核内的定位,而细胞质是无色的。

2. 植物细胞

（1）取材与固定:取洋葱鳞茎表皮数片置于盛有 10% 甲醛的培养皿内,固定 15min。取出标本放入含蒸馏水的小烧杯中,用吸管吸取蒸馏水反复冲打标本,然后吸弃蒸馏水,该步骤重复 3 次。

（2）三氯醋酸处理:在含有标本的烧杯内注入 5% 三氯醋酸 30ml 充分浸泡,然后将烧杯放在电炉上加热,使烧杯内溶液的温度保持 90℃,处理 15min。弃去处理液,反复用自来水冲洗标本至无三氯醋酸气味。

（3）染色:取一半标本移入另一烧杯内,两烧杯内标本分别用 20ml 0.1% 酸性固绿染液（pH 2.0）和 20ml 0.1% 碱性固绿染液（pH 8.0）染色 1~5min;然后吸弃染液,用胶头吸管吸取 pH 2.2 和 pH 8.0 的磷酸氢二钠 - 柠檬酸缓冲液各 20ml,吹洗 30s。

取出两烧杯内标本,放在载玻片上,分别加一滴 pH 2.2 和 pH 8.0 的磷酸氢二钠 - 柠檬酸缓冲液,用解剖针展平,加盖玻片。

（4）镜检:0.1% 酸性（pH 2.0）固绿染液染色的标本,酸性蛋白质染成绿色;0.1% 碱性（pH 8.0）固绿染液染色的标本,碱性蛋白质染成绿色。请根据两种染色液染色标本的观察结果,比较酸性蛋白质和碱性蛋白质在细胞内的分布情况。

（二）细胞骨架蛋白

1. 洋葱表皮细胞

（1）取材:切开洋葱鳞茎,撕取中层鳞片的内表皮,剪成 2~3mm² 大小的小片,浸入装有 5ml 6mmol/L PBS（pH 6.5）的小烧杯中,处理 5~10min,使其下沉。

（2）抽提:吸弃 PBS,加入 3ml 1%TritonX-100,置 37℃恒温水浴箱内处理 20~30min,提取细胞骨架以外的蛋白质。

（3）洗涤:吸弃 1%TritonX-100,再用 3ml M- 缓冲液轻轻洗涤 3 次,每次 5min,使细胞骨架稳定。

（4）固定:吸弃 M- 缓冲液,加入 5ml 3% 戊二醛,固定 15~20min。

（5）洗涤:吸弃固定液,用 5ml 6mmol/L PBS（pH 6.5）洗涤 3 次,每次 5min。最后用吸水吸去残液。

（6）染色:滴加 5 滴 0.2% 考马斯亮蓝 R250 染液染色 3~5min。

（7）制片:吸弃染液,用蒸馏水洗涤 2~3 次,将标本取出平铺在载玻片上,在标本上加盖玻片。

（8）镜检:光镜下可见洋葱表皮细胞的轮廓,细胞内存在着被染成蓝色、粗细不等的纤

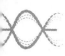

维网络结构,即为细胞骨架的微丝束。有的细胞中核的周围还可见到一些放射状分布的细丝。选择染色较好的细胞,转换高倍镜观察,可见细胞骨架的立体结构。

2. 人口腔黏膜上皮细胞

(1)涂片:用牙签刮取人口腔黏膜上皮细胞,置于装有生理盐水的试管中,洗涤离心 1~2 次,留取剩约 0.5ml 沉淀,用吸管将其吹打均匀制成细胞悬液,然后将细胞悬液滴在玻片上制备涂片并晾干。

(2)漂洗:晾干的涂片用 M- 缓冲液漂洗 3 次。

(3)抽提:将细胞涂片置于盛有 1% Triton X-100 的玻璃染色缸中,室温或 37℃处理 20~30min。

(4)漂洗:从 1% Triton X-100 中取出涂片,用 M- 缓冲液漂洗 3 次,每次 3min。

(5)固定:用吸水纸吸去涂片上多余的 M- 缓冲液,将涂片放入含有 3% 戊二醛固定液的玻璃染色缸内,固定 10~15min。

(6)洗涤:取出涂片,用吸水纸吸去多余固定液,然后用磷酸盐缓冲液(pH7.2)洗涤 3 次,每次 3min;最后用吸水纸吸去残液。

(7)染色:在涂片上滴加 5 滴 0.2% 考马斯亮蓝 R250 染液,染色 30~60min。吸弃染液,小心用蒸馏水冲洗数次。

(8)镜检:在涂片的标本上加盖玻片,然后将涂片置显微镜下观察。低倍镜下可见细胞质中微丝组成的应力纤维呈紫蓝色,沿细胞长轴平行或交叉分布;细胞核圆形,呈浅蓝色,位于细胞近中央,核内可见 2~5 个深蓝色的核仁。选择结构典型的细胞换用高倍镜进一步观察。

【分析思考】

1. 显示细胞内蛋白质酸碱性质的原理是什么?
2. 酸性蛋白和碱性蛋白染色的原理是什么?
3. 说明着色的碱性蛋白可能是什么物质?
4. 在显示细胞中酸性蛋白与碱性蛋白的实验中,为何所用固绿染液的 pH 不同?

【实验报告】

1. 绘图表示蟾蜍红细胞中酸性蛋白质及碱性蛋白质在细胞内的分布。
2. 绘图表示洋葱表皮细胞与人口腔黏膜上皮细胞的细胞骨架分布。

三、糖的细胞化学

【目的要求】

1. 熟悉多糖的细胞化学反应原理。
2. 掌握细胞中多糖的细胞化学染色方法。

【实验原理】

糖的细胞化学是利用多糖的显色反应原理显示细胞内多糖的存在与分布的细胞化学染色方法。

1. 过碘酸希夫反应 糖类中的单糖,在组织标本固定、脱水和包埋等组织化学操作过程中会被抽提掉,因此,一般组织化学标本片上所能显示的糖类主要是多糖,包括糖原、中性黏多糖、糖蛋白和糖脂等。动物摄入机体的糖类大部分转变为脂肪,储存在脂肪组织内,只有一小部分以糖原形式储存,在机体需要葡萄糖时,糖原可迅速分解。糖原是以糖苷键相连的多葡萄糖分子组成的聚合体,有"动物淀粉"之称,主要贮存于肌肉细胞和肝细胞中。

过碘酸希夫反应(periodic acid Schiff reaction,PAS 反应)是由 McManus 于 1946 年在 Feulgen 反应的基础上发展而来,是显示糖原和其他多糖物质最经典,也是最直接的细胞化学方法。在该反应中,强氧化剂过碘酸先将多糖中葡萄糖的乙二醇基(CHOH—CHOH)氧化成两个游离醛基(—CHO);然后,游离醛基再与 Schiff 试剂反应生成不溶性紫红色复合物,附着在多糖存在的部位,复合物颜色的深浅与多糖含量成正比。

2. 淀粉的显色反应　淀粉是植物细胞中储存的多糖,遇碘液呈蓝色,加热时蓝色消失,冷却后蓝色又重新出现。淀粉有直链淀粉和支链淀粉之分,蓝色物质是直链淀粉遇碘生成的不稳定的碘化淀粉。

【实验用品】

（一）材料

小鼠肝脏石蜡切片、新鲜马铃薯。

（二）器材

显微镜、载玻片、盖玻片、镊子、双面刀片、吸水纸、培养皿、毛笔等。

（三）试剂

1% 碘液。

【实验步骤】

（一）PAS 反应

PAS 染色的小鼠肝脏切片观察:取 PAS 染色的小鼠肝脏切片在光镜下观察,可见肝细胞略呈多角形,中央有 1~2 个染成蓝色的细胞核,细胞质中可见许多紫红色的糖原颗粒(图 3-1)。缓慢移动标本,可见肝细胞中糖原颗粒数量不等,形态大小也不尽相同,有的呈细小颗粒状,有的呈较大块状。切片上位于组织周边的肝细胞,其糖原颗粒往往偏于细胞一侧(与边界相对的一侧),呈半月形,以致组织周边糖原分布呈覆瓦状。这是制片过程中,固定液渗入将糖原颗粒冲挤到细胞一侧所致,并不代表生活状态下细胞内糖原的分布情况。此外,在糖原颗粒之间,还可以看到大小不一、未被染色的空泡,这是制片过程中脂肪滴被脂溶性溶剂溶解所致。

（二）淀粉显色反应

1. 徒手切片

（1）将马铃薯切成切面约 0.5cm×0.5cm、长 2~3cm 的小段,削平切面,以便徒手切片。取一培养皿,备好清水。

（2）用左手大拇指和示指夹住条状马铃薯,使之固定不动;为防止刀伤,拇指应略低于示指,并使马铃薯上端超出示指 2~3mm。

（3）徒手切片前,先在刀口上蘸些水,起滑润作用。右手大拇指和示指捏住刀片的右下角,刀口向内,并与马铃薯切面平行。

（4）左手保持不动,以右手上臂带动前臂,使刀口自外侧左前方向内侧右后方拉切。连续切下数片备用。

注意:徒手切片时,只用臂力而不要用腕力或指关节的力量;两手不要紧靠身体或压在桌子上,动作要敏捷;要一次切下,中途不要停顿,切忌作"拉锯"式切割。切片过程中,刀口和材料要不断蘸水,以保持刀口锋利,并避免材料失水变形。徒手切片的关键是要切得薄而厚度均匀。

2. 染色 选择切得薄而均匀的马铃薯片,移至载玻片上,滴加 1% 碘液 1 滴,可见其立即被染成蓝色,随即加盖玻片。溢出的碘液用吸水纸沾吸。

3. 镜检 镜下观察,可见在多角形的薄壁细胞中,有许多染成蓝色的椭圆形淀粉粒(图3-2),染色浅的淀粉粒上可见清晰的脐与轮纹。

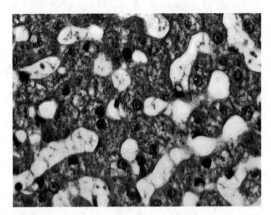

图3-1 PAS染色的小鼠肝组织(示肝细胞内糖原颗粒)

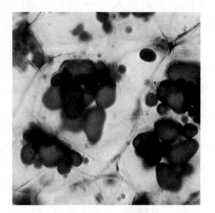

图3-2 马铃薯块茎薄壁细胞(示淀粉粒)

【分析思考】

1. 动植物细胞中糖类物质有哪些?其中的主要储能物质分别是什么?
2. 显示动物细胞内糖原的原理是什么?
3. 为什么遇碘变蓝色的淀粉,加热时蓝色消失,冷却后又重新出现?

【实验报告】

1. 绘图表示肝细胞中糖原的分布,并标出糖原颗粒。
2. 绘出 2~3 个马铃薯薄壁细胞,并标出淀粉颗粒和细胞壁。

实验 4 细胞的显微结构

【目的要求】

1. 熟悉光学显微镜下细胞器的形态及其在细胞内的分布。
2. 熟悉线粒体、液泡系的超活染色原理及方法。
3. 掌握光镜下线粒体、液泡系在细胞内的分布。

【实验原理】

超活染色,又称体外活体染色,是对从机体获取的尚处于存活状态的组织或细胞进行的体外染色方法。用作超活染色的染色剂具有专一性,无毒或毒性较小,不影响或较少影响细胞的生命活动,对细胞和组织不产生任何物理变化和化学变化。

1. 线粒体超活染色 碱性染料詹纳斯绿 B(Janus green B)是线粒体的专一性活体染色剂,毒性较小,具有脂溶性,能穿过细胞质膜及线粒体膜进入线粒体,并通过其结构中带正电荷的染色基团结合到带负电荷的线粒体内膜和嵴膜上。线粒体是细胞内能量代谢的重要场所,含有多种与能量代谢有关的酶类。其中内膜和嵴膜上的细胞色素氧化酶可使结合的詹纳斯绿 B 始终保持氧化状态而呈蓝绿色(有色状态),而线粒体周围细胞质中的詹纳斯绿 B 则被还原为无色的色基(无色状态)。

2. 液泡系超活染色 动物细胞内,由单层膜形成的泡状结构属于液泡系(线粒体和核膜除外),包括高尔基体、溶酶体、内质网、胞饮体和吞噬体等。弱碱性染料中性红(neutral red)是液泡系的专一性活体染色剂,只将活细胞中的液泡系染成红色,而细胞核、线粒体和胞质溶胶完全不着色。中性红的染色机制可能与液泡系含有特定蛋白质有关。软骨细胞内含较多的糙面内质网和发达的高尔基体,能合成分泌软骨黏蛋白及胶原纤维等,液泡系发达,因此,液泡系的超活染色常以软骨组织为材料。

3. 高尔基体银染 高尔基体是 1898 年,意大利科学家 C·Golgi 在用银染法对神经细胞染色时发现的。由于高尔基体的嗜银性,重铬酸钾与硝酸银反应生成的黑色或棕褐色铬酸银沉淀,沉积于神经元中。

4. 中心体龙胆紫染色 中心体周围的中心粒周物质起微管组织中心的作用,微管组织中心的 γ 微管蛋白环状复合物(γ-TuBC)就像一粒种子,可与 α/β 微管蛋白异二聚体结合,即具有成核作用,微管由此生长、延长。采用碱性染料龙胆紫对细胞分裂期的染色体进行染色时,可以清晰地看到细胞的中心体。

【实验用品】

(一)材料

家兔、蟾蜍、小鼠肾脏切片、兔脊神经节银染切片、马蛔虫子宫龙胆紫染色切片。

(二)器材

解剖器械、解剖盘、培养皿、载玻片、盖玻片、吸管、吸水纸、注射器(处死兔子用)、显微镜、擦镜纸、香柏油(或液体石蜡)、无水乙醇(或乙醚乙醇混合液)。

(三)试剂

1/300 詹纳斯绿 B 染液(兔用、两栖类用)、0.80%Ringer 液(兔用)、0.65%Ringer 液(两栖类用)、1/3 000 中性红染液(两栖类用)。

【实验步骤】

(一)细胞显微结构切片观察

1. 线粒体(小鼠肾脏切片) 低倍镜下,可见许多圆形和椭圆形的环状结构,这是横切面的肾小管。切面上肾小管由一层紧密排列的上皮细胞围成,细胞呈锥形,但轮廓不清。换高倍镜或油镜进一步观察,可见肾小管上皮细胞细胞质中有许多染成蓝黑色的短杆状或颗粒状的结构,即线粒体。通常,细胞基部胞质中线粒体分布较多(图 4-1)。

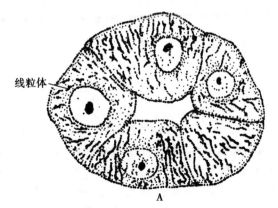
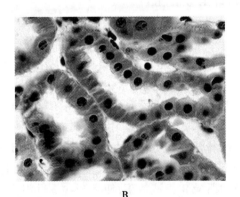

A   B

图 4-1 肾小管细胞中的线粒体

A. 模式图;B. 显微结构图。

线粒体

2. 高尔基体（兔脊神经节切片）　低倍镜下,染成棕黄色的神经纤维束将神经节细胞(卵圆形或圆形)分隔成群;换高倍镜观察,可见神经节细胞中央着色较淡,呈浅黄色或空泡状,此为细胞核所在部位。有的神经节细胞的核中心可见黄褐色、折光较强的核仁,核周围细胞质被染成淡黄色,其中有染成黑色或棕褐色的弯曲线状、网状、颗粒状结构,即为高尔基体(图4-2)。细胞核周围的细胞质被染成浅黄色,其中有棕色的弯曲线形、网状和颗粒状结构,即高尔基体

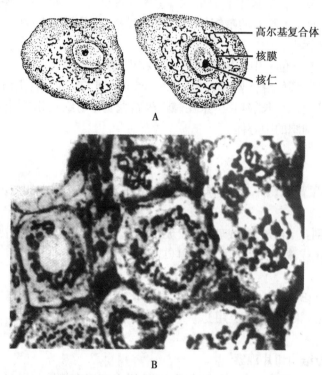

图 4-2　脊神经节细胞中的高尔基体

A. 模式图；B. 显微结构图。

3. 中心体（马蛔虫子宫切片）　低倍镜下,马蛔虫子宫腔内有许多由受精卵膜围成的大腔,即围卵腔,腔内有处于不同分裂期的受精卵细胞。在分裂中期的受精卵细胞内,可见深蓝色条状的染色体排列在赤道板上,染色体两侧的细胞两极,各有一个染成深蓝色的小颗粒——中心粒;中心粒与周围较致密的中心粒周物质合称为中心体。高倍镜下,可见到中心体外围有放射状的星射线,在两中心体之间还可观察到由许多微管构成的纺锤体(图4-3)。

（二）超活染色

1. 线粒体超活染色

（1）取材和染色:用空气栓法处死家兔,将家兔腹面向上置于解剖盘内,迅速打开腹腔,在兔肝脏边缘切取一小块肝组织($2\sim5mm^3$),放入盛有 0.80%Ringer 液的培养皿内;用镊子轻轻挤压肝组织,洗去血液,然后用镊子夹取肝组织放于载玻片上,并在肝组织上滴加 1/300 詹纳斯绿 B 染液数滴,使组织块下部浸入染液中,上部露在染液外面,使细胞内的细胞色素氧化酶可以在有氧条件下充分进行氧化反应(线粒体着色),直至组织块边缘染成蓝绿色,通常需要染色 30min。

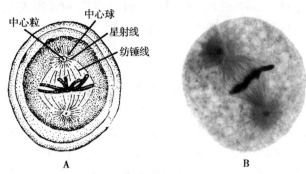

图 4-3 马蛔虫受精卵有丝分裂中期（示中心体）

A. 模式图；B. 显微结构图。

本实验也可用蟾蜍肝脏，不同之处在于洗去蟾蜍肝脏血液用 0.65%Ringer 液；染色方法、染色时间同上。

（2）制片：染色后，先用剪刀将组织块剪碎；再用镊子按压肝组织块，此时会有一些细胞或细胞团与组织块分离；移去稍大的组织块，使分离下来的细胞或细胞团留在载玻片上；在载玻片上加一滴 0.80%Ringer 液（兔肝）或 0.65%Ringer 液（蟾蜍肝），盖上盖玻片，吸去多余水分。

（3）镜检：光镜下可见兔肝细胞细胞核周围散布一些染成蓝绿色的短杆状或圆形颗粒状结构，即为线粒体。蟾蜍肝细胞中的线粒体则被染成蓝绿色，呈颗粒状，细胞核周围分布较多。

2. 液泡系超活染色

（1）取材：以捣毁脊髓法处死蟾蜍，剪开胸腹腔，暴露剑突，在剑突软骨的边缘剪下一小片，放在载玻片上。

（2）染色：在载玻片的标本上滴 2 滴 1/3 000 中性红染液，染色 15min 后用吸水纸吸去染液，加 1 滴 0.65%Ringer 液，盖上盖玻片，吸去多余的 Ringer 液。

（3）镜检：光镜下观察，可见软骨细胞为椭圆形，细胞核周围的细胞质中有许多染成玫瑰红色、大小不一的小泡，即为软骨细胞液泡系。

【分析思考】

1. 线粒体、液泡系超活染色的原理是什么？
2. 简述线粒体、高尔基体的显微结构特征。
3. 简述超活染色的兔（或蟾蜍）肝细胞和蟾蜍剑突软骨细胞的显微结构特征。
4. 观察银染兔脊神经节切片时，为什么有的神经节细胞核中见不到核仁？

【实验报告】

1. 绘鼠肾小管细胞结构图。
2. 绘兔脊神经节细胞结构图。
3. 绘线粒体超活染色的蟾蜍肝细胞结构图。

实验 5 细胞的生理活动

【目的要求】

1. 了解纤毛和鞭毛的结构特点及运动方式。

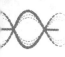

2. 了解细胞质膜对物质通透性的一般规律,溶血与细胞质膜通透性的关系。

3. 通过观察动物红细胞在不同溶液中的溶血现象,加深理解细胞质膜的选择通透性及溶血发生的机制。

【实验原理】

细胞的生理活动包括细胞运动、细胞质膜的物质运输、细胞内物质代谢和能量代谢、细胞增殖和分化、细胞对外界环境的反应、肌肉细胞收缩、神经细胞兴奋的传导等。本实验通过对细胞运动及细胞质膜通透性现象的观察,从而对细胞的生理活动有初步的认识。

1. 细胞运动 纤毛和鞭毛是单细胞和多细胞生物细胞表面伸出的具有运动功能的杆状特化结构。通常将多而短的称纤毛,少而长的称鞭毛,它们都能推动细胞向前运动。纤毛和鞭毛由纵行排列的微管束构成的轴丝外被细胞质膜构成,纵向由基体和杆状部两部分组成,基体埋在细胞内,杆状部突出于细胞表面。纤毛和鞭毛各段轴丝的微管构成不同,中段轴丝的微管呈 9×2+2 结构,即周边 9 组二联微管(A 管和 B 管)和两条中央微管。二联管通过 A 管动力臂(ATP 酶)分解 ATP 分子,释放能量,使二联管之间产生滑动,通过二联管与中央微管辐射丝的连接,把滑动转变成弯曲,引起纤毛和鞭毛的运动。

蟾蜍呼吸道黏膜上皮细胞纤毛的协同摆动,能推动流质和固体颗粒从其表面通过。精子尾部与纤毛和鞭毛的结构相似,精细胞中的远端中心粒演变为精子的轴丝,轴丝也为 9×2+2 结构,是精子的运动器官。

2. 细胞质膜的通透性 细胞质膜是一种半透膜,对物质的通透有选择性。将红细胞置于低渗溶液中时,由于细胞内的渗透压高于细胞外,所以水分子很快进入细胞内,使细胞胀破,发生溶血,混浊的红细胞悬液会变成红色透明的血红蛋白液;将红细胞置于不同溶质的等渗溶液中时,红细胞质膜对各种溶质分子的通透性不同,因此溶质分子渗入细胞内的速度也不同,由此导致红细胞内渗透压增高、水分摄入、细胞质膜破裂而出现溶血的时间也不同。细胞质膜对物质的通透性与物质的分子量、脂溶性及是否带电荷等有关。据此,可通过测量溶血时间来估计细胞质膜对各种物质通透性的大小。

【实验用品】

(一)材料

雄蟾蜍、家兔。

(二)器材

显微镜、香柏油(或液体石蜡)、无水乙醇(或乙醚乙醇混合液)、擦镜纸,解剖器械,蜡盘、大头针、牙签、载玻片、盖玻片、培养皿、吸管、吸水纸、蜡屑、烧杯、试管、试管架、50ml 注射器、5ml 注射器、硫酸纸。

(三)试剂

0.17mol/L 氯化钠溶液、0.17mol/L 氯化铵溶液、0.17mol/L 醋酸铵溶液、0.17mol/L 硝酸钠溶液、0.12mol/L 草酸铵溶液、0.12mol/L 硫酸钠溶液、0.32mol/L 葡萄糖溶液、0.32mol/L 甘油、0.32mol/L 乙醇、0.32mol/L 丙醇、0.27mol/L 氯化钠溶液、无菌肝素(500U/ml)、生理盐水、蒸馏水。

【实验步骤】

(一)蟾蜍上颌黏膜上皮细胞的纤毛运动

1. 取雄蟾蜍 1 只,以捣毁脊髓法处死;将蟾蜍腹部向上,展开四肢,用大头针固定在蜡盘上。

2. 沿蟾蜍两侧口角向后剪开口腔两侧壁约 1cm，将下颌翻转固定在腹部，暴露出咽头（图 5-1）。

3. 在上颌中线距喉头 1cm 处放置蜡屑，观察蜡屑是否运动、向什么方向移动。思考蜡屑为什么能移动。记录蜡屑从开始移动到消失的时间。

4. 用眼科剪剪取上颌喉头前部黏膜约 2mm×2mm 的小块，用牙签挑取黏膜块，将纵切面贴于载玻片上；加 1 滴生理盐水于标本上，加盖玻片。

5. 镜检　在低倍镜下找到有纤毛运动的部位，换用高倍镜，仔细观察纤毛的运动规律。

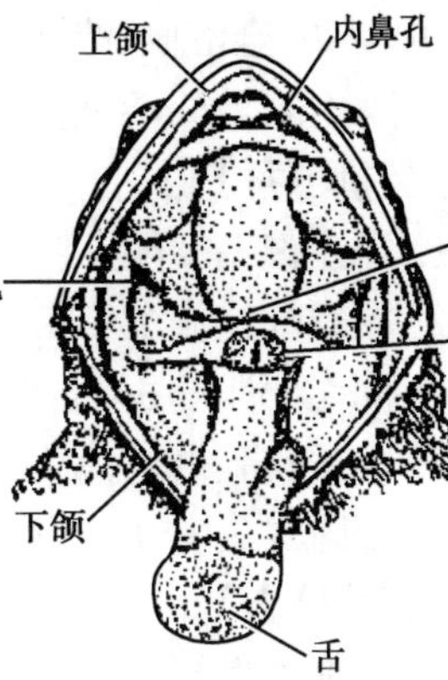

图 5-1　蟾蜍口腔内面图

（二）蟾蜍精子的鞭毛运动

1. 将已处死的雄蟾蜍沿腹中线剪开胸腹腔壁，暴露出黄色圆柱状精巢。

2. 剪取精巢放入盛有生理盐水的培养皿中，用镊子夹住其一端在水中摆动，洗去血污。

3. 把洗净的精巢移到一干净的培养皿中，用眼科剪将精巢充分剪碎，加入数滴生理盐水混匀。

4. 用吸管吸取培养皿内液体，滴 1 滴在载玻片上，盖上盖玻片，2~3min 后镜检。

5. 镜检　用低倍镜观察（把光线调暗些），可见视野中有许多运动的精子。选择运动缓慢的精子，换用高倍镜或油镜观察。蟾蜍精子由头部、颈部和尾部构成。头部呈长锥形，颈部极短（有前、后中心粒，不易看到）。尾部细长，有时可见波浪状的边缘，主要由轴丝构成。轴丝的结构似鞭毛，精子靠尾部弯曲、摆动而运动。

（三）细胞质膜的通透性

1. 制备 10% 兔红细胞悬液　先在烧杯中加入生理盐水 45ml。用空气栓塞处死法处死家兔，剪开家兔胸廓，暴露心脏；吸取 500U/ml 无菌肝素 0.5ml 湿润 5ml 注射器针筒，抽取兔心脏内血液至 5ml，注入烧杯中，轻轻振摇，混匀，制备成 10% 兔红细胞悬液。兔红细胞悬液外观表现为红色不透明液体。

2. 红细胞在不同渗透压溶液中的变化

（1）每组（2 人）取 3 支试管，依次编号为 1 号（低渗）、2 号（等渗）、3 号（高渗）。首先在三支试管内加入 0.3ml 的 10% 红细胞悬液，然后在 1、2、3 号试管内分别加入蒸馏水、0.17mol/L 氯化钠溶液和 0.27mol/L 氯化钠溶液各 3ml。用硫酸纸封住管口，倒置一次。分别观察红细胞在低渗、等渗和高渗溶液中的溶血现象（溶液的颜色变化、溶液是否透明等），记录观察结果。

（2）用牙签分别蘸取上述试管的低渗、等渗和高渗溶液各一滴于载玻片上，盖上盖玻片，在显微镜高倍镜下所观察到的低渗、等渗和高渗溶液中的兔红细胞形态有何不同？

3. 测定各种物质对红细胞质膜的通透性　取试管 10 支，依次编号。各管中分别加入准备好的 10 种等渗溶液 2ml，再分别加入 10% 兔红细胞悬液 0.2ml，轻轻摇动混匀。以低渗溶血管为对照，观察各管溶液颜色变化，并记录溶血时间，分析不同溶液造成溶血时间差异的原因。

4. 溶血的判断标准

（1）不溶血：液体分两层，上层浅黄色透明，下层红色不透明。

（2）不完全溶血：溶液浑浊，上层变成红色。

（3）完全溶血：溶液变红且透明。

【分析思考】

1. 简述鞭毛、纤毛结构及运动机制。

2. 在蟾蜍上颌黏膜上皮细胞的纤毛运动实验中，蜡屑为什么能移动？如何移动？从蜡屑开始移动到消失用多长时间？

3. 根据实验结果，说明脂溶性大小对细胞质膜通透性的影响。

4. 不同溶液中红细胞溶血时间有何不同？为什么？

【实验报告】

1. 分别绘出等渗和高渗状态下的兔红细胞形态。

2. 列表并分析兔红细胞通透性的实验结果。

实验6　细胞的超微结构

【目的要求】

通过观看视频资料、观察电镜照片，掌握各种细胞器的超微结构特征，加深对相关理论知识以及细胞超微结构与功能关系的理解。

【实验原理】

超微结构，又称亚显微结构，是指超出光学显微镜分辨水平，在电子显微镜（简称电镜）下才能观察到的细胞结构的统称。电子显微镜的分辨率远高于光学显微镜，能分辨细胞内的各种细胞器，细胞表面结构和各种细胞连接，也能分辨细菌〔含纳米细菌〕、支原体和病毒等各种病原微生物。

按结构和用途，电子显微镜可分为透射电子显微镜、扫描电子显微镜、反射电子显微镜和发射电子显微镜，其中透射电子显微镜（transmission electron microscope，TEM）和扫描电子显微镜（scanning electron microscope，SEM）最常用。透射电子显微镜常用于观察普通光学显微镜不能分辨的细微结构，扫描电子显微镜主要用于观察标本表面的形貌。

【实验用品】

视频资料、电镜照片。

【实验步骤】

（一）播放细胞超微结构视频资料

（二）观察细胞超微结构电镜照片，辨认细胞各部分的超微结构

【内容提要】

（一）细胞质膜

人红细胞质膜（plasma membrane）的电镜照片上，可见位于细胞最外缘的质膜呈三层结构，内外两层为电子密度较高的致密层（深色），两层之间为电子密度较低的疏松层（浅色），总厚度为 7.5~10nm（图 6-1）。除细胞质膜外，细胞器的界膜也具有此三层结构，此种结构称为单位膜（unit membrane）。

（二）细胞核

细胞核（nucleus）大多位于细胞的中央（图 6-2），包括核膜、染色质、核仁和核基质等几部分。

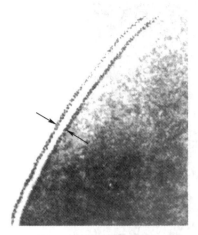

图 6-1　质膜的超微结构

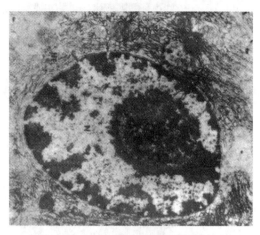

图 6-2　细胞核的超微结构

1. 核膜　电镜下,核膜(nuclear membrane)由内核膜、外核膜两层单位膜及二者之间的核周隙构成。注意:不要将此结构误认为单位膜的三层结构。外核膜外表面有颗粒状核糖体附着,并与内质网相连,核周隙与内质网腔相通。内核膜、外核膜融合形成均匀分布的核孔,核孔是细胞核与细胞质之间物质交换的通道。

观察两栖动物肠上皮细胞电镜照片和胚胎间叶细胞冷冻断裂蚀刻复型电镜照片显示的核膜脂双层断面的结构。

2. 染色质　染色质(chromatin)是分裂间期细胞核内能被碱性染料着色的物质,根据其形态和功能分为两类:常染色质(euchromatin)和异染色质(heterochromatin)。着色较深、形态各异、大小不等的颗粒状或块状结构是异染色质。在异染色质之间,着色较浅、结构较疏松的细颗粒状或细丝状结构是常染色质。

观察两栖动物肠上皮细胞和豚鼠浆细胞电镜照片显示的染色质结构。

3. 核仁　电镜下,核仁(nucleolus)是无膜包被的纤维丝网状结构,由纤维中心、致密纤维中心和颗粒组分 3 个不完全分隔的特征性区域构成。纤维中心是 rRNA 基因——rDNA的存在部位,表现为低电子密度的斑状浅染区,被核仁中电子密度最高的环形或半月形致密纤维组分包围。颗粒组分位于核仁的外周,颗粒直径 15~20nm,含有处于不同加工阶段的核糖体亚基前体颗粒。颗粒组分是核仁的主要结构,核仁的大小主要是颗粒组分决定的。包围在核仁周围的异染色质称为核仁结合染色质,伸入核仁内纤维中心的常染色质称为核仁染色质。

观察豚鼠腺泡电镜照片显示的是细胞核中核仁的结构。

4. 核基质　核基质(nuclear matrix)充填于染色质及核仁间隙中,为电子密度低的无定形物质,位于核仁中的核基质也称为核仁基质。

（三）内质网

根据膜外表面是否附有核糖体,将内质网(endoplasmic reticulum)分为糙面内质网和光面内质网。糙面内质网呈扁平囊状,互相连通,构成膜性管道系统;电镜下,可见膜色深、腔色浅,膜外表面附着颗粒状的核糖体。光面内质网呈分支小管和小泡状,有的彼此相连成网,膜表面光滑,无核糖体附着(图 6-3)。

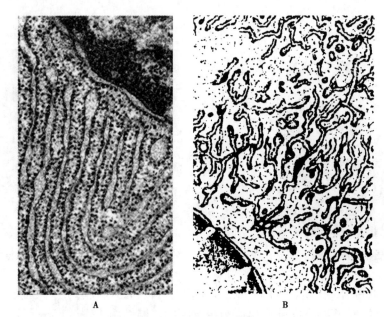

图 6-3　内质网的超微结构

A. 糙面内质网；B. 光面内质网。

　　观察蝙蝠腺泡细胞、小鼠肝细胞电镜照片上糙面内质网，人肾上腺皮质细胞电镜照片上光面内质网的结构。

（四）高尔基体

　　高尔基体（Golgi body）是由单位膜形成的、不同形态的囊泡状结构构成（图 6-4），囊泡结构包括扁平囊、大囊泡和小囊泡。扁平囊是高尔基体最显著部分，通常由 4~8 层弯曲成弓形的扁平囊泡重叠构成，其囊腔狭窄；扁平囊有凸、凹两面：凸面又称形成面，面向细胞质和内质网；凹面又称成熟面（分泌面），靠近细胞质膜，凹面可扩大成大泡（大囊泡）。大囊泡分布于成熟面，由成熟面迁移而来，含有分泌蛋白逐渐浓缩形成的分泌颗粒。小囊泡见于形成面，由附近的糙面内质网芽生而来。

　　观察大鼠睾丸精原细胞、附睾细胞电镜照片上的高尔基体结构。

（五）溶酶体

　　溶酶体（lysosome）是由单层单位膜围成的球形小体，内含多种酸性水解酶（图 6-5）。电镜下，内容物的电子密度均匀的溶酶体为初级溶酶体（primary lysosome）；内容物的电子密度不均匀者为次级溶酶体（secondary lysosome），是正在进行消化作用的溶酶体。溶酶体功能状态及消化的内容物不同，有不同的名称，如含有未被消化的残存物质的残余体，含有线粒体残骸的自噬溶酶体等均属次级溶酶体。电镜下要注意区分溶酶体与线粒体，溶酶体内无嵴，电子密度高。

　　观察大鼠肝细胞电镜照片，细胞质中电子密度高、内部无嵴的圆形或椭圆形结构是初级溶酶体；观察小鼠回肠细胞电镜照片上的多囊体。

（六）过氧化物酶体

　　过氧化物酶体（peroxisome）是由一层单位膜围成的圆形或椭圆形细胞器，一般比溶酶体小，内含中等电子密度的颗粒物质。观察大鼠肝细胞和人肝细胞过氧化物酶体，电镜下，大鼠肝细胞中过氧化物酶体呈球形，由单层膜包被，内部无嵴，电子密度低，内有一个深色的类

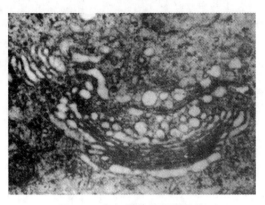

图 6-4　高尔基体的超微结构

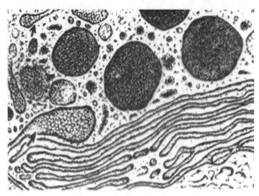

图 6-5　溶酶体的超微结构

核体。类核体是尿酸氧化酶的结晶,人的肝细胞过氧化物酶体没有类核体。请将过氧化物酶体与线粒体、溶酶体的形态、结构进行比较。

(七) 线粒体

线粒体(mitochondrion)是由双层单位膜包围而成的封闭结构(图 6-6)。内膜和外膜之间的腔隙称为膜间隙(或外腔),内膜向内折叠形成板状或管状的嵴,内膜围成的腔称为基质腔(或内腔)。内膜、外膜与嵴膜呈深色的线状结构,嵴膜和内膜上附着有许多深色的球形小体——基粒;膜间隙和基质腔内物质的电子密度较低,色浅;基质中含有电子密度很高的基质颗粒。在负染电镜照片上,可清晰地看到内膜上由球部、柄和基片 3 部分构成的白色基粒。

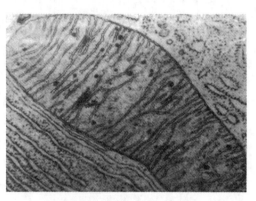

图 6-6　线粒体的超微结构

(八) 核糖体

核糖体(ribosome)由大、小两个亚基组成,无单位膜包被。附着在糙面内质网的核糖体称为附着核糖体,游离于细胞质中的核糖体称为游离核糖体;多个核糖体附着在一个 mRNA 分子链上构成多核糖体。

电镜下,核糖体呈颗粒状,电子密度高,颜色很深;小鼠肝细胞电镜照片上,糙面内质网膜上有许多颜色很深的颗粒状结构,即附着核糖体;胞质中多核糖体成簇分布,呈螺旋状、念珠状,还可见到 5~8 个甚至更多的核糖体被一条线状的 mRNA 分子串在一起的放大图像。经负染技术处理且放大 400 000 倍的电镜照片上,80S 核糖体色浅,可区分核糖体的大、小亚基。

(九) 中心粒

中心粒(centriole)是中心体的主要构成成分,为圆筒状小体。构成中心体的中心粒,成对存在、互相垂直,圆筒的壁由 9 组纵行排列的三联微管组成。电镜下,中心粒纵切面上颜色较深的管状结构是组成中心粒的微管;横切面上,可见每个中心粒由 9 组三联微管组成,每组 3 根斜行排列的微管形如风车的叶片。

观察鸡胚的胎膜腺细胞电镜照片上构成中心体的中心粒结构。

（十）微管和微丝

微管（microtubule）为中空的管状结构，外径为24~26nm，分散存在于细胞质中；微丝（microfilament）为实心纤维状结构，直径为5~6nm，常成束平行排列在细胞质膜下，也有的分散并交织成网状（图6-7）。

观察大鼠肾小球细胞电镜照片上微管和微丝的纵切面。

（十一）细胞全貌

观察大鼠肝细胞电镜照片。

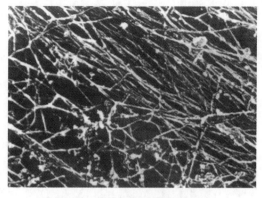

图6-7 微管和微丝的超微结构

【分析思考】

电镜下各种细胞器的超微结构特点如何？各有何功能？

【实验报告】

观察领取的电镜照片，在对应表格上，以打钩方式标出指示部位超微结构名称。

实验7 细胞分裂

【目的要求】

1. 掌握有丝分裂各期的细胞形态结构变化特点。
2. 掌握减数分裂的基本过程及各期的形态特征。
3. 掌握减数分裂前期Ⅰ各亚期、中期Ⅰ和中期Ⅱ的染色体形态特点。

【实验原理】

细胞通过分裂而增殖，生物体通过细胞分裂，达到个体生长与繁衍的目的。

有丝分裂是真核细胞的主要增殖方式。细胞分裂过程中细胞核形态发生显著变化，专门执行细胞分裂功能的临时性细胞器——有丝分裂器，能确保把已复制好的两套遗传物质平均分配给2个子细胞，故此种细胞分裂方式称为有丝分裂。根据形态学特征，可将有丝分裂连续的变化过程分为前期、中期、后期和末期4个阶段。

减数分裂是有性生殖个体生殖细胞形成过程中特有的细胞分裂方式，包括2次连续的分裂过程。由于染色体只在第一次减数分裂（减数分裂Ⅰ）前复制一次，而第二次减数分裂（减数分裂Ⅱ）前不复制，因此，减数分裂最终产生的4个配子细胞的染色体都只有减数分裂前细胞中染色体数目的一半，故此种细胞分裂方式称为减数分裂。

减数分裂过程与有丝分裂基本相同，主要区别在于减数分裂Ⅰ的前期（前期Ⅰ）历时长，染色体形态变化复杂，是减数分裂过程中最具特征的时期。根据染色体形态特点，可把前期Ⅰ分为5个亚期：细线期、偶线期、粗线期、双线期和终变期。

蝗虫染色体数目较少，便于观察、操作简便，取材方便，因此，蝗虫是研究动物细胞减数分裂的理想材料。蝗虫体细胞、初级卵母细胞及初级精母细胞有常染色体11对，雌蝗虫有2条X染色体（XX），雄蝗虫只有1条X染色体（XO），故雌蝗虫有24条染色体（2n=22+XX），雄蝗虫有23条染色体（2n=22+XO）。在减数分裂生成生殖细胞过程中，雌蝗虫形成的卵细胞都具有12条染色体（n=11+X）；雄蝗虫形成的精细胞，11条染色体（n=11+O）和12条染色体（n=11+X）两种类型各占一半。

【实验用品】

（一）材料

预处理的洋葱根尖、马蛔虫子宫横切片、雄蝗虫精巢压片。

（二）器材

镊子、载玻片、盖玻片、吸水纸、显微镜、香柏油（或液体石蜡）、无水乙醇（或乙醚乙醇混合液）、擦镜纸。

（三）试剂

改良的苯酚品红染液、Carnoy 固定液、1mol/L HCl 溶液（60℃预热）、95% 乙醇、85% 乙醇、70% 乙醇、蒸馏水。

【实验步骤】

一、有丝分裂

（一）植物细胞

1. 洋葱根尖压片的制备

（1）根尖处理：待根长达 2cm 时，切下根尖，浸入 Carnoy 固定液中 4h，在 95% 和 85% 乙醇中各 30min，最后在 70% 乙醇中保存（实验课前完成）。

（2）水解：取出根尖放在载玻片上，滴加少量 1mol/L HCl 溶液（60℃）于根尖上，水解 8min，蒸馏水水洗 3 次。

（3）染色与压片：切取根尖的乳白色分生区，用镊子轻轻地捣碎，滴 1 滴改良苯酚品红染液，染色 20min 后，盖上盖玻片。在盖玻片上面覆盖一张吸水纸后，先用拇指垂直压，再用一手指按住盖玻片的一端，另一手用铅笔橡皮头轻轻敲打，使细胞压成均匀的薄层（敲打时，勿使盖玻片移动）。

2. 根尖细胞有丝分裂标本的观察　取根尖压片，先在低倍镜下找到根尖末端，从根尖末端往上依次为根冠区、生长区、延伸区和根毛区（图 7-1）。选择根尖较前端生长区观察，可见细胞呈四方形、染色较深，紧密排列成行。缓慢移动标本，选择细胞分裂旺盛的部位，换高倍镜观察，可见许多处于不同分裂期的细胞（图 7-2）。细胞周期各期的结构特点如下（图 7-3）：

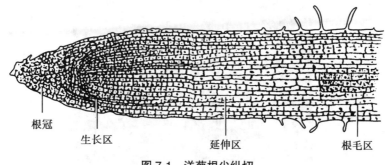

图 7-1　洋葱根尖纵切

（1）间期：间期细胞较小，细胞核清晰可见，染色质分布较均匀，细胞核中可见 1~2 个核仁。

（2）前期：细胞核膨大，染色质细纤丝状并盘曲呈网状；前期末，染色质逐渐螺旋形成细

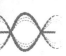

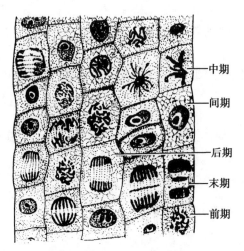

图 7-2　根尖细胞的有丝分裂

中期
间期
后期
末期
前期

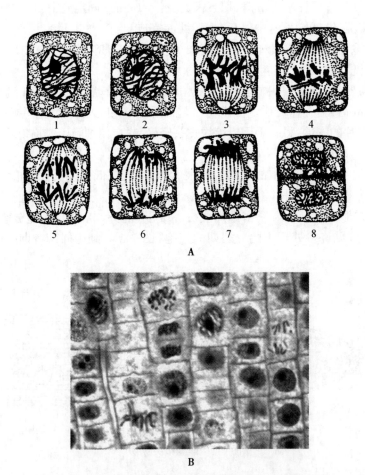

1　2　3　4

5　6　7　8

A

B

图 7-3　洋葱根尖细胞有丝分裂的前期、中期、后期和末期
A. 模式图;B. 显微结构图。

线状的染色体,分散于细胞质中。核仁、核膜消失,纺锤丝出现。每条线状的染色体由两条姐妹染色单体组成。

（3）中期:细胞开始伸长,所有染色体向细胞中央移动,形成赤道板;中期染色体最粗,结构最清晰。此时,来自两极的纺锤丝与染色体的着丝点相连,构成纺锤体(光镜下不易见到)。

（4）后期:细胞拉得更长,两条姐妹染色单体在着丝粒处纵裂,彼此分开;由于纺锤丝的牵引,分开的两条染色单体移向两极。此期染色体多呈 V 形,V 形的尖端为着丝点。

（5）末期:移到两极的染色单体解旋为染色质,纺锤体消失,核膜、核仁重新出现,形成 2 个细胞核。在两个新细胞核之间的细胞中央,高尔基体小囊泡融合成细胞板,进而形成细胞壁,分隔细胞质,形成 2 个子细胞。

（二）动物细胞

取马蛔虫子宫横切片,先用低倍镜观察,可见子宫腔内有许多处于不同发育阶段的圆形或椭圆形受精卵细胞。每个受精卵细胞的周围都有一层厚而染色淡的卵壳,注意不要把卵壳误认为是细胞质膜。受精卵细胞在卵壳内分裂,受精卵细胞与卵壳之间有宽大的围卵腔。在有些受精卵细胞的表面或卵壳的内面可见有极体附着。选择处于有丝分裂不同阶段的受精卵细胞,转换高倍镜仔细观察有丝分裂各期细胞的结构特征(图 7-4)。

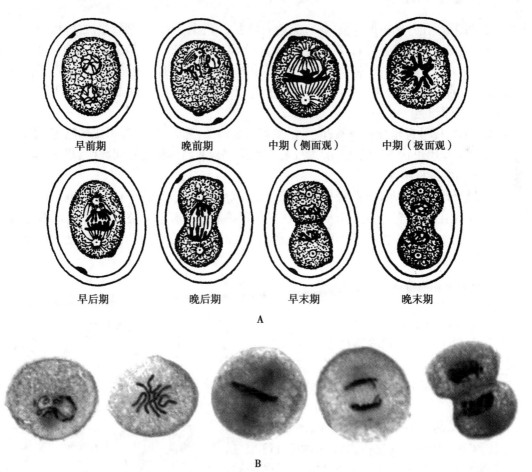

图 7-4　马蛔虫受精卵有丝分裂过程
A. 模式图;B. 显微结构图。

1. 间期　细胞质内有两个近圆形的细胞核,一为雌原核,另一为雄原核。两个原核形态相似不易分辨,核内染色质分布比较均匀,核膜、核仁清楚,细胞核附近可见中心粒存在。

2. 前期　细胞核膨大,复制后的一对中心体彼此分离,向细胞两极移动;中心粒周围出现辐射状星射线(即电镜下的星体微管);细胞核中染色质逐渐浓缩形成染色体;核仁、核膜消失。在切片标本上,染色体呈细丝状、点状或短棒状,无规则地分散在胞质中;由于切面不同,有时只见到一个中心体或见不到中心体。

3. 中期　两中心体移到两极,纺锤体形成,染色体位于纺锤体中央。在切片标本上,极面观可见染色体(共6条)放射状排列如菊花样;侧面观,两极各有一个中心体,染色体呈"一"字排列。精细调焦,可见纺锤丝与染色体着丝粒相连。

4. 后期　姐妹染色单体在着丝粒处分离,数目相同的2组子染色体在纺锤丝牵引下,移向细胞两极。镜下可见,染色单体的着丝粒向着细胞一极,两臂朝向细胞中部,形成V形。两组染色体像两把相对的梳子分别向两极移动。后期末,细胞中部质膜出现横缢凹陷。

5. 末期　到达两极的染色单体解旋变成染色质,纺锤体和星射线消失,核仁、核膜重新出现,细胞质膜的横缢凹陷加深,最后缢缩形成2个子细胞。

二、减数分裂

雄蝗虫精巢压片标本的观察:雄蝗虫精巢是由多条圆柱形的精细管组成,蝗虫精子发生于精细管上皮。精细管有两端,盲端游离,另一端(附着端)开口于输精管。在制作良好的压片上,从游离的盲端起始,可依次看到精原细胞、精母细胞、精细胞及精子等。先在低倍镜下分清精细管的不同位置,然后换用高倍镜或油镜,根据细胞结构,辨认细胞类型及所属时期。

(一)精原细胞

精原细胞通过有丝分裂增殖,位于精细管的游离端,胞体较小,圆形或椭圆形,核大,染色深,染色质呈团块状不规则排列。每个精原细胞都含有与体细胞相同数目的染色体。

(二)初级精母细胞

初级精母细胞由精原细胞经过生长期分化发育而成,染色体数与精原细胞相同。每个初级精母细胞经过减数分裂Ⅰ形成2个次级精母细胞。与有丝分裂过程相似,减数分裂Ⅰ也可分成前、中、后、末4期;所不同的是,前期Ⅰ历时长,细胞核的变化复杂,是减数分裂最有特征性的阶段。

1. 前期Ⅰ　依细胞核内染色体的形态变化,前期Ⅰ又可分为下列各亚期:

(1)细线期(leptotene):染色质凝集成细长的线状染色体,且绕成一团,故细胞核大染色浅,难以分辨。在细丝状的染色体上,可见念珠状的染色粒。核内也可见到核仁(图7-5)。此期标本镜下特点为:染色体呈细丝状或绒毛状,色淡。

(2)偶线期(zygotene):此期细胞核更大,染色体形态与细线期变化不大,仍细而长;各对同源染色体开始从一端配对,配对的一端聚集于细胞核的一侧,另一端则散开,形成花束状。配对的结果形成11个四联体,四联体也

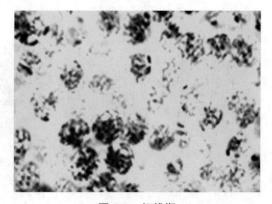

图7-5　细线期

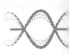

称为二价体。X 染色体因无法配对而异固缩成为 X 小体,存在于核膜内缘。由于此期存在时间较短,通常难以观察到。此期标本镜下特点为:染色体细长,线条多,有时可清晰看到两条同源染色体的某些片段并排在一起(图 7-6)。

(3)粗线期(pachytene):配对的同源染色体(四联体)缩短变粗,整个核内染色体显得稀疏(图 7-7)。此期非姐妹染色体单体间可发生交换,故看到交叉现象。此期标本镜下特点为:染色体呈粗线条状,线条粗短,常可见染色粒。

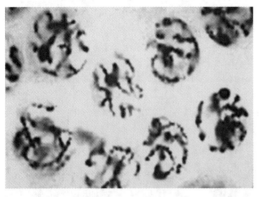

图 7-6　偶线期

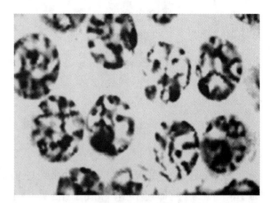

图 7-7　粗线期

(4)双线期(diplotene):染色体变得更为粗短,表面不光滑,似绒毛状。可区分出 11 个四联体和 1 个 X 染色体。四联体的 2 条同源染色体结合紧密,不易分清其中的每条染色体。同源染色体开始分离,但因同源染色体的非姐妹染色体单体间的交叉存在而分离不完全。交叉是非姐妹染色体单体间局部交换的表现。随着交叉逐渐端化,可看到染色体上有一点或两点交叉在一起,呈 X、O 或 ∝ 等各种图像(图 7-8)。X 染色体呈棒状,无交叉。此期标本镜下特点为:染色体较粗线期更浓缩、粗短,可见较大的环状、"8"字形及杆状等形态的染色体,而且环状染色体的环大而细。

(5)终变期(diakinesis):染色体浓缩得更为粗短,表面光滑,形态多种多样,多分布于核的四周。四联体清晰可数。交叉进一步端化,形成 O、V、X、Y 等特殊图像。核仁、核膜消失(图 7-9)。

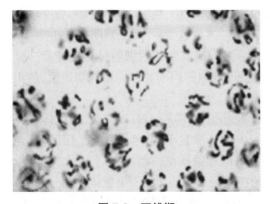

图 7-8　双线期

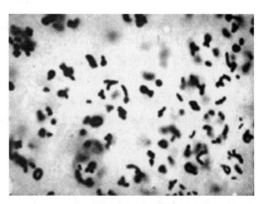

图 7-9　终变期

2. 中期Ⅰ　四联体高度浓缩,边缘光滑,排列在细胞中央,侧面观呈板状,极面观呈空

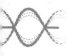

心花状。核膜完全消失,纺锤体出现,着丝粒与纺锤丝相连(图7-10)。

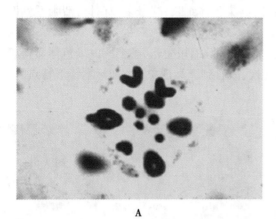

A

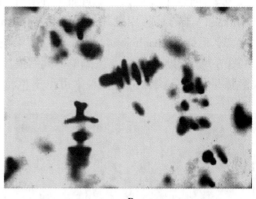

B

图 7-10　减数分裂中期 Ⅰ

A. 极面观;B. 侧面观。

3. 后期 Ⅰ　四联体的 2 条同源染色体分开,非同源染色体随机组合成 2 组,其中 1 组为 11 条染色体,另 1 组为 12 条染色体;受纺锤丝的牵引,2 组染色体分别移向两极(图7-11)。极面观,染色体在两极排成菊花形。此期标本镜下特点为:可见到两组 V 形染色体。

4. 末期 Ⅰ　到达两极的染色体解旋为染色质,核仁、核膜重新形成;细胞拉长,中部缢缩使胞质均分,形成 2 个体积较小的二分体,即次级精母细胞。

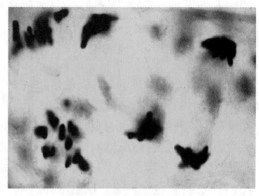

图 7-11　减数分裂后期 Ⅰ

(三)次级精母细胞

第一次减数分裂完成形成的两个次级精母细胞,分别含有 11 条和 12 条染色体,即染色体数目已减半($n=11+X$,或 $n=11+0$)。

1. 间期 Ⅱ　第一次减数分裂生成的次级精母细胞即处于间期,且间期极短,不进行 DNA 复制,直接进入第二次减数分裂。减数分裂 Ⅱ 也分为前、中、后、末 4 期,其形态变化与体细胞有丝分裂的分裂期相似,但从细胞形态上看,染色体数目少一半,细胞明显变小。

2. 前期 Ⅱ　染色体显示分开的趋势,像花瓣状排列,使前期 Ⅱ 的细胞呈实心花状。核仁、核膜消失。此期也非常短暂。由于雄蝗虫次级精母细胞的间期 Ⅱ 和前期 Ⅱ 均短暂,故不易观察到。甚至有可能从末期 Ⅰ 直接进入中期 Ⅱ。

3. 中期 Ⅱ　纺锤体再次出现。侧面观,染色体在赤道面排成一列;极面观,染色体像花朵在细胞中央排成一圈(图7-12)。与中期 Ⅰ 相比,中期 Ⅱ 细胞小,染色体也细小,其形态与有丝分裂中期染色体相似。镜下往往看到两个中期 Ⅱ 细胞紧挨在一起。

4. 后期 Ⅱ　由于纺锤丝的牵引,各染色体着丝粒纵裂形成的 2 组子染色体(染色单体),分别移向细胞两极;每组有 n 条($n=11$ 或 12)子染色体,其数目是初级精母细胞(23 条)的一半(图7-13)。此期标本镜下特点为:可见到两组棒状的子染色体。

5. 末期 Ⅱ　移到两极的两组子染色体,解螺旋并聚集成团,形成染色质;核膜、核仁重

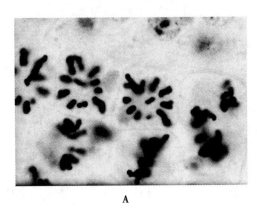
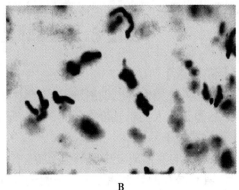

图 7-12 减数分裂中期Ⅱ
A.极面观;B.侧面观。

新出现,形成新细胞核,进而形成2个圆形的精细胞。镜下可见精细胞比次级精母细胞更小,细胞核较大(图7-14);有时可见4个紧挨的精细胞,即由1个初级精母细胞经减数分裂Ⅰ和减数分裂Ⅱ,最后形成的4个精细胞,其中2个含11条子染色体,另2个含12条子染色体。减数分裂形成的4个子细胞也称为四分体。至此,减数分裂Ⅱ完成。

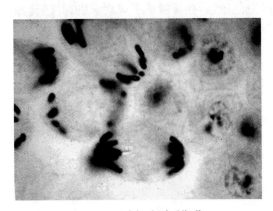

图 7-13 减数分裂后期Ⅱ

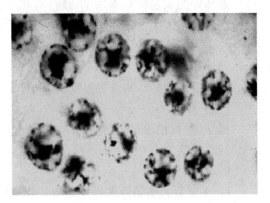

图 7-14 精细胞的形态

(四)精子

精细胞先由圆形变为圆头长尾形,以后逐渐变为椭圆头长尾形,最终形成细长纺锤形的头部和长尾部的精子(sperm)(图 7-15)。

【分析思考】

1. 比较初级精母细胞、次级精母细胞与精细胞中染色体、染色单体及DNA分子的数目。

2. 比较减数分裂与有丝分裂的异同点。

【实验报告】

1. 绘出有丝分裂间期、前期、中期(极面观、侧面观)、后期和末期细胞结构图各一个。

2. 绘出雄蝗虫精母细胞减数分裂前期Ⅰ双线期和终变期、中期Ⅰ、中期Ⅱ的细胞分裂象图各一个。

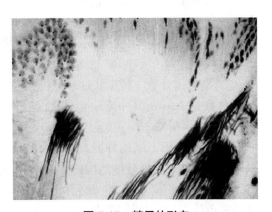

图 7-15 精子的形态

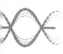

实验 8　人类非显带染色体核型分析

【目的要求】

1. 熟悉人外周血淋巴细胞培养、染色体标本制备的原理。

2. 熟悉正常人类非显带染色体核型特征及核型分析方法。

【实验原理】

人外周血的有形成分中,只有白细胞有细胞核,而白细胞中只有淋巴细胞(主要是小淋巴细胞)具有潜在的分裂能力。在细胞进入分裂期时,间期细胞核中的染色质逐渐折叠压缩形成染色体;在分裂期的中期,染色体表现为短而粗的典型结构。

外周血淋巴细胞培养液中加入有丝分裂刺激剂植物血凝素(PHA),可使处于 G_0 期、具有潜在分裂能力的淋巴细胞转化为具有分裂能力的淋巴母细胞,淋巴母细胞进入细胞周期。在细胞培养进入对数生长期时,在培养液中加入纺锤体抑制剂秋水仙碱,可使处于分裂过程的淋巴细胞停滞在分裂中期;收获细胞时,用 0.075mol/L KCl 溶液对细胞进行处理,0.075mol/L KCl 溶液的低渗作用使细胞膨胀,滴片时细胞质膜容易破裂,染色体均匀分散;经离心、固定、制片等过程,最终可获得便于观察分析的染色体标本。

制备好的染色体标本片,不经特殊处理,直接染色,然后在显微镜下观察识别,并进行核型分析的过程称为染色体非显带核型分析。

【实验用品】

(一)材料

人类染色体标本制备视频资料、非显带染色体标本片、非显带染色体核型照片。

(二)器材

显微镜、香柏油(或液体石蜡)、无水乙醇(或乙醚乙醇混合液)、擦镜纸,废液缸、剪刀、镊子、胶水、牙签。

【实验步骤】

(一)观看人类染色体标本制备视频资料

(二)观察非显带染色体标本片

取非显带染色体标本片,先在低倍镜下观察;选择染色体形态较好、分散均匀,无细胞质背景的中期分裂象,换油镜仔细观察。按显微镜下看到的染色体图像,在实验报告纸上描绘出染色体分布的快速线条图(图 8-1),在图中,应尽可能体现各染色体的原有方位、相对长度及着丝粒位置。

1. 染色体计数　依据快速线条图计数染色体,确定有无数目异常。人类正常体细胞的染色体数是 2n=46,其中常染色体 22 对,性染色体 1 对,正常男性核型表达为 46,XY,女性核型表达为 46,XX。

2. 染色体形态结构分析　每条染色体含有 2 条染色单体,通过着丝粒彼此连接。自着丝粒向两端伸展的染色体结构称染色体臂,染色体臂分为短臂(用 p 表示)和长臂(用 q 表示)。

根据着丝粒位置,人类染色体分为 3 类:中着丝粒染色体,长臂与短臂几乎相等;近中着丝粒染色体,长臂与短臂能明显区分;近端着丝粒染色体,短臂极短,着丝粒几乎在染色体的顶端,有时短臂上能看到随体。

在油镜下观察染色体的形态结构、次缢痕的位置,以及有无断裂、缺失、重复、易位、倒

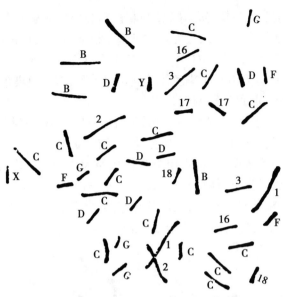

图 8-1　染色体分布的快速线条图

位、环状染色体和等臂染色体等染色体结构畸变。根据非显带染色体的形态结构特征,在快速线条图的各染色体旁标出染色体的组号或序号。观察非显带染色体时,能够准确区分的染色体序号包括 1、2、3、16、17、18 和 Y 染色体。

(三)非显带染色体核型照片剪贴分析

为确定被检个体有无染色体数目或结构异常,常在显微镜下寻找最佳中期分裂象,进行显微摄影并放大照片;将照片上每条染色体剪下,依据人类细胞遗传学命名的国际体制(ISCN),按照染色体的大小和着丝粒的位置等特征,将染色体贴在核型分析表的相应位置上。此过程称为染色体核型照片剪贴分析,简称核型分析。

ISCN 将人类染色体分成 A、B、C、D、E、F 和 G 7 个组,各组所包含的染色体及染色体的结构特征见表 8-1。

表 8-1　人类非显带染色体结构特征

组号	序号	大小	着丝粒类型	随体	说明
A	1、3	最大	中着丝粒	无	3 号比 1 号略小;1 号长臂近着丝粒处常见次缢痕
	2		亚中着丝粒		
B	4、5	次大	亚中着丝粒	无	与 C 组相比,B 组短臂较短
C	6~12、X	中等	亚中着丝粒	无	9 号、10 号、12 号短臂较短;X 大小介于 7 号、8 号之间;9 号长臂近侧常见次缢痕
D	13~15	中等	近端着丝粒	有	各号长度相似,难以区分
E	16	小	中着丝粒	无	18 号较 17 号短臂更短些;部分个体长臂近着丝粒处可见次缢痕
	17、18		亚中着丝粒		
F	19、20	次小	中着丝粒	无	难以区分
G	21、22	最小	近端着丝粒	有	两长臂常呈分叉状,二者难以区分
	Y			无	两长臂常并拢

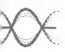

染色体核型分析按照计数染色体总数、判断性别和照片剪贴的顺序进行。如染色体数目正常且无明显结构异常,可初步认为为正常核型。根据 G 组染色体的特征,如最小的近端着丝粒染色体(G 组)是 5 条(2 条 21 号、2 条 22 号和 1 条 Y 染色体),可判断为男性;如 G 组是 4 条,则为女性。用剪刀将每条染色体连同组号剪下,将每组染色体按照大小顺序依次排列,此时如发现排列有误,可进行调整。

在非显带染色体核型照片剪贴前,先根据各组染色体的结构特征,依次辨认出 A、B、D、E、F、G 组染色体,剩余的则确定为 C 组染色体;然后在每条染色体旁用铅笔标出组号。用剪刀将每条染色体连同组号剪下,将每组染色体按照大小顺序依次排列,此时如发现排组有误,可进行调整;最后,将染色体组号剪去,将各号染色体排在染色体核型分析表的相应位置上,用胶水贴牢。粘贴时,应使染色体的短臂居上、长臂居下,并使着丝粒在一条直线上(图 8-2、图 8-3)。剪贴过程要细心,防止丢失染色体。

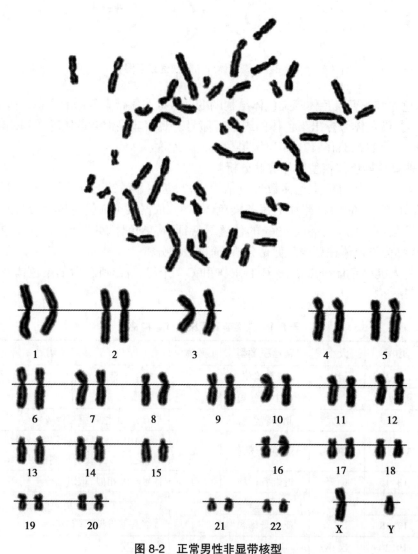

图 8-2　正常男性非显带核型

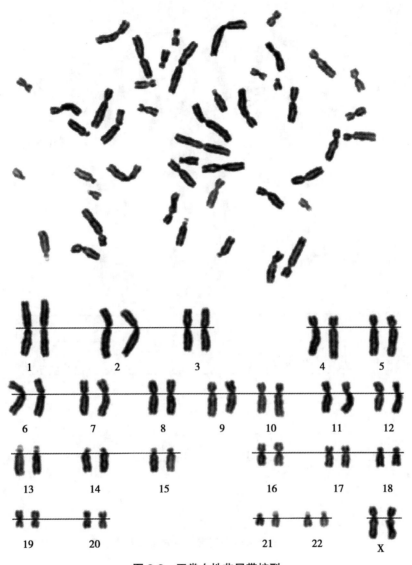

图 8-3 正常女性非显带核型

（四）染色体测量

用直尺测量核型分析表中每号染色体的短臂长度和长臂长度,计算每一染色体的相对长度、臂比和着丝粒指数。

（1）臂比 = 长臂长度 / 短臂长度。

（2）着丝粒指数 =（短臂长度 / 染色体全长）× 100%。

（3）相对长度 =[每一条染色体的长度 / 该细胞单倍体染色体（22+X）总长度]× 100%。

【分析思考】

1. PHA 和秋水仙碱在淋巴细胞培养过程中各有何作用?

2. 收获细胞时,用 0.075mol/L KCl 溶液处理细胞的作用是什么?

【实验报告】

1. 绘出显微镜下非显带染色体快速线条图（染色体旁标注染色体号数或组号）。

2. 正常女性非显带染色体核型剪贴分析（图 8-4,见文末插图 8-5）。

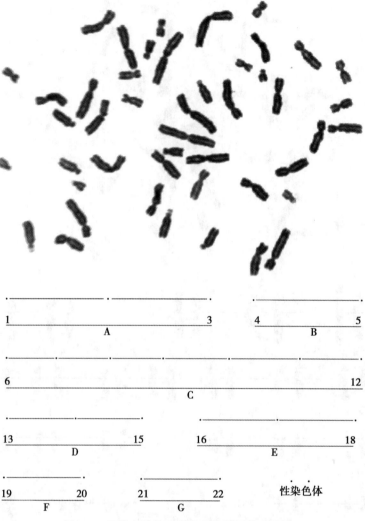

图 8-4　正常女性非显带染色体核型剪贴分析

实验 9　细 胞 培 养

【目的要求】

1. 了解哺乳动物细胞原代培养、传代培养及冻存的基本方法和操作过程。

2. 熟悉用倒置相差显微镜观察培养细胞的形态和生长状况。

3. 初步掌握细胞培养的无菌操作技术。

【实验原理】

细胞培养(cell culture)是从体内取出组织或细胞,在体外模拟体内生理环境,在无菌、适当温度和一定营养条件下,使之生存、生长、繁殖并维持其结构和功能的技术。细胞培养在生命科学理论研究和应用科学研究中广泛应用,在分子生物学研究、细胞工程及基因工程等高科技领域也不可或缺。

体外培养的细胞根据其生长方式的特点可分为贴附型与悬浮型两大类。能附着于底物(支持物)表面生长的细胞属贴附型细胞,形态上大体分为上皮细胞型和成纤维细胞型。大多数活体细胞在体外培养的条件下,均呈现出贴附型生长的特点;有些细胞在培养时可悬浮于培养液中生长,而不需贴附于支持物上,此类细胞即为悬浮型细胞。悬浮型细胞(包括取自血液、脾脏和骨髓的细胞,尤其是白细胞及血液系统肿瘤细胞)悬浮生长良好,显微镜下观察细胞呈圆形。

在进行正常细胞培养时,不论细胞的种类和供体的年龄如何,在细胞生存过程中,大致都经历原代培养期、传代期和衰退期3个阶段。

1. 细胞的原代培养 从供体取得组织或细胞至第一次传代之前的体外细胞培养阶段即为原代培养(primary culture),也叫初代培养。原代培养的细胞主要特点是组织和细胞刚刚离体,其生物学性状尚未发生较大变化,仍具有二倍体遗传特性,被广泛应用于药物测试、细胞分化等实验研究中;而且,原代培养的细胞具有在体细胞的某些特性,可用于某些特殊实验研究,如原代软骨细胞适合软骨细胞膜片培养,进而可分析软骨细胞膜片的成软骨性能。

组织块法和消化法是最基本和最常用的原代培养方法。组织块法是将刚离体的,有旺盛生长活力的组织剪成小块,接种于含培养液的培养瓶,培养瓶中的培养液及培养条件可根据不同细胞生长的需要做适当调整。新生细胞大约24h后可从贴壁的组织块边缘生长,继而分裂繁殖。组织块法操作简便,培养的细胞较易存活,在对来源有限、数量少的组织进行原代培养时,首选组织块法。消化法应用胰蛋白酶、胶原酶等将已剪切成小块组织中妨碍细胞生长的间质(包括基质、纤维等)消化,使组织中原本结合紧密的细胞连接松散、相互分离,形成含单细胞或细胞团的悬液,从而很快得到大量活细胞。活细胞在培养瓶中能在短时间内生长成片。虽然消化法的原代细胞产量高,但步骤烦琐、易污染,一些消化酶价格昂贵,实验成本高,仅适用于培养大量组织。

2. 细胞的传代培养 原代细胞培养过程中,单层培养细胞相互汇合,当增殖达到一定数量后,会因生存空间不足或密度过大,产生接触抑制或者营养耗竭,从而导致生长受影响。因此,必须对细胞及时分离、稀释。细胞由原培养瓶内分离稀释后再接种到新的培养瓶的过程称为传代(passage)。原代细胞传代后即为细胞系,以后可继续传代。

细胞自接种至新培养皿中至其下一次再接种传代的时间为细胞的一代。每代细胞的生长过程可分为三个阶段,先进入增殖缓慢的滞留阶段,以后为增殖迅速的指数增殖期(适宜进行各种试验),最后到达增殖停止的平台期,传代过晚将影响下一代细胞的生长增殖。

根据不同细胞,培养细胞传代采取不同的方法。大多数贴壁生长的细胞用消化法传代,通常是利用一些消化剂(常用 0.25% 胰蛋白酶)首先使贴壁细胞与培养器皿表面及其他细胞间发生分离,然后进行稀释、再培养;部分贴壁生长但贴附不牢固的细胞也可用直接吹打传代;悬浮生长的细胞可以采用直接吹打或离心沉淀后再分离传代,或直接用自然沉降法吸除上清液后,再吹打传代。

3. 细胞的冻存 细胞冻存是将细胞储存在低温环境中,减少细胞代谢,实现长期储存的一种技术。培养细胞的传代及日常维持过程中,其各种生物学特性会逐渐发生变化,并随着传代次数的增加和体外环境条件的改变而不断有新的变化,同时培养器皿、培养液等也被大量地消耗,适当的操作和合适的冻存条件可以减少细胞特性的改变或丢失,起到细胞保种的作用。目前细胞冻存已成为细胞培养室的常规工作和通用技术,从增殖期到形成致密的单层细胞以前的培养细胞都可以用于冻存,但最好为对数生长期细胞。

冻存细胞的基本原则是控制降温速率,缓慢冷冻。细胞在不加任何保护剂的情况下直接冷冻会导致细胞内、外的水分迅速形成冰晶,进而对细胞结构与功能造成一系列的损害,如机械损伤、蛋白质变性、电解质升高等,最后可引起细胞死亡。为了避免细胞内冰晶的形成,在冻存细胞时常向培养液中加入适量在深低温冷冻后对细胞无明显毒性的二甲基亚砜(DMSO)或甘油,其相对分子质量较小而溶解度大,易穿透进入细胞中,使细胞内冰点下降,并可提高细胞质膜对水的通透性,再配合以缓慢冷冻的方法,可使细胞内的水分逐步地渗透出胞外,避免了冰晶在细胞内大量的形成,从而减少由于冰晶形成所造成的细胞损伤。因此,正确且成功的冻存对细胞的长久应用起着非常重要的作用。

【实验用品】

(一)材料

新生大鼠或细胞系(如 U251 细胞、HeLa 细胞、MGC80-3 细胞、K562 细胞等)。

(二)器材

超净工作台、CO_2 培养箱、倒置相差显微镜、水浴箱、高压蒸汽消毒锅、超低温冰箱、液氮罐、离心机、解剖器械、眼科剪刀、消毒器械包、酒精灯、离心管、移液管、烧杯、大平皿、培养皿(消毒)、冻存管(1~2ml)、96 孔培养板、不锈钢滤网(100 目、200 目)、血细胞计数板、培养瓶、弯头吸管、移液器、枪头、盖玻片。

(三)试剂

DMEM 培养液、0.25% 胰蛋白酶、D-Hanks 液 /PBS(磷酸缓冲盐溶液)、小牛血清、0.4% 锥虫蓝、双抗(青霉素和链霉素)、75% 乙醇、2% 聚维酮碘、二甲基亚砜。

【实验步骤】

(一)原代培养

1. 组织块法(以新生大鼠心肌细胞的原代培养为例)

(1)处死动物:取出生 2~3d 新生乳鼠 1 只,颈椎脱白法或剪断颈动脉放血法处死,浸入75% 乙醇烧杯 2~3s 后取出,置于大平皿中移入超净工作台。

(2)取材:打开消毒器械包,用 2% 聚维酮碘和 75% 乙醇消毒胸腹部,用解剖剪打开胸腔,取出心脏置于消毒的培养皿中,吸管吸取灭菌 D-Hanks 液 /PBS 反复冲洗 3 次,去除血细胞。为避免杂细胞污染,需用解剖镊将心脏组织块上所附的结缔组织尽可能去除。

(3)剪切:将心肌组织移入另一消毒的培养皿中,沿纵轴剪开,用眼科剪刀剪成 0.5~$1mm^3$ 的小块,加 2~3 滴 DMEM 培养液轻轻吹打,使组织块悬浮于培养液中。

(4)接种:用弯头吸管端部分次吸取组织块到培养瓶中,要避免吸得过高,组织块黏附于吸管壁而丢失。用弯头吸管头移动组织块,使其均匀分布于培养瓶底部,组织块间距控制在 0.5cm 左右,数量为 20~30 块 / 培养瓶(25ml)。组织块放置好后,轻轻将培养瓶翻转,让瓶底朝上,吸取 2~3ml 培养液(液层厚约 15mm),沿培养瓶颈缓缓滴入,培养液的量以恰好能浸润组织块底部,但不会使组织块漂浮为佳。盖好瓶盖,将培养瓶倾斜放置在 37℃的 CO_2培养箱培养。

(5)培养:培养 2~4h,待组织块贴附后,将培养瓶慢慢翻转平放,静置培养。此过程动作要轻,让液体缓缓覆盖组织块。动作过快液体产生冲力可使黏附在培养瓶底的组织块漂起而造成原代培养失败。

(6)观察:移动培养瓶时尽量使培养液震荡撞击组织块,倒置相差显微镜观察到有少量细胞从组织块周围游离而出时,根据培养液颜色,补加或更换培养液,培养液表面如有漂浮的组织块,要及时吸弃(图9-1)。

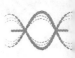

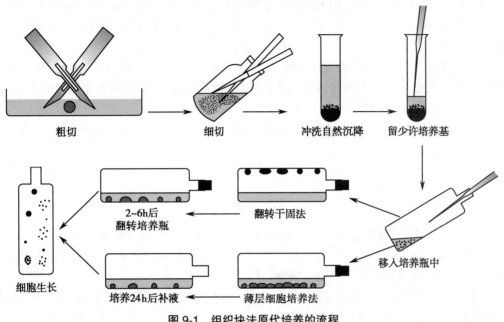

图 9-1 组织块法原代培养的流程

2. 消化法（以胰蛋白酶消化为例）

（1）处死动物、取材及剪切：同组织块法。

（2）消化：心肌组织块用 D-Hanks 液 /PBS 漂洗至液体澄清，移入无菌离心管，静置使组织块自然沉到管底，弃上清；再注入 5~10 倍组织量的 0.25% 胰蛋白酶，混匀后加盖无菌塞密封，置 37℃水浴消化 20~30min，每 5min 摇动 1 次。当组织块变疏松、颜色略白时，取出离心管于超净工作台内吸弃消化液，加 2~3ml 培养液终止消化。

（3）分散组织块：吸管反复吹打至大部分组织块分散成单细胞或细胞团，将收集的细胞悬液用 100 目、200 目的不锈钢滤网过滤至烧杯中，除掉未消化充分的大块组织。

（4）计数及稀释：取过滤液 1ml，用血细胞计数板计数。根据计数结果用培养液稀释，稀释后的细胞密度以（3~5）× 10^5 个 /ml 为宜。

（5）接种培养：将稀释好的细胞悬液分装于培养瓶中，一般 25ml 小方瓶分装 4~5ml，青霉素瓶分装 1ml。培养瓶上做好标记，瓶盖旋紧后再松半个螺旋，37℃的 CO_2 培养箱培养。

（6）观察：接种培养后每日观察培养液颜色变化及细胞生长状况。培养液黄色且混浊表示污染，紫红色表明细胞生长不良，橘红色表明细胞生长良好。培养 3~4d 时，若培养液变黄、澄清，表明细胞生长，但营养成分不足，代谢产物堆积，可更换 1/2 新培养液或维持液。此后，每 3~4d 更换新培养液或维持液。

（二）传代培养

1. 贴壁细胞的传代培养

（1）准备：从培养箱中取出原代培养的细胞，显微镜观察确定生长良好且适宜传代后备齐实验用品，连同培养瓶放入超净工作台。

（2）消化：用吸管吸出培养瓶内的原培养液，加入适量 PBS，轻轻摇动清洗，以除去细胞表面悬浮碎片，弃清洗液。加 2~3ml 消化液（0.25% 胰蛋白酶），以覆盖整个细胞培养面为宜。培养瓶置室温或培养箱内 2~3min 后，在倒置显微镜下观察，若细胞回缩近球形且相互间不再连成片,或翻转培养瓶肉眼观察发现细胞单层出现针孔大小的缝隙,则迅速吸出消化液,加入新配制的培养液约 3ml 于培养瓶中终止消化;如果未见空隙,说明消化程度不够,可将消化时间稍延长。

（3）稀释及分装:用吸管吸取培养液,反复冲击瓶壁上的细胞,直至全部细胞被冲下,轻轻混匀制成细胞悬液。取细胞悬液计数并用 0.4% 锥虫蓝染色,计算细胞密度及细胞活力并补加适量培养液稀释,调整细胞密度为 5×10^4 个 /ml 后分装于 2 瓶或多瓶中。如原培养瓶为 5ml 培养液,分装 2 瓶时需补加培养液到 10ml,混匀后分一半到另一培养瓶。分装好的培养瓶需标明日期、细胞代号等。

（4）培养与观察:轻轻摇动分装好的培养瓶,置 37℃ 的 CO_2 培养箱培养。每日观察培养液的颜色及细胞生长状况。

2. 悬浮细胞的传代培养

（1）离心传代:取培养瓶于超净工作台内吸管吹打、制悬,将细胞悬液转移到无菌离心管,800~1 000r/min 离心 8~10min,弃上清,加适量新配制的培养液吸管吹打、制悬,细胞计数、稀释、分装、培养及观察等操作同贴壁细胞的传代培养。

（2）直接传代:让悬浮细胞缓慢沉淀到瓶底,弃上清 1/2~1/3,吸管吹打、制悬,细胞计数、稀释、分装、培养及观察等操作同贴壁细胞的传代培养。

（三）细胞的冻存

1. 配制冻存液　取已抽滤的,含 10%~20% 小牛血清的培养液 90ml,用一次性注射器向培养液中加入 10ml 二甲基亚砜（DMSO）或已消毒的甘油,吸管混匀。

2. 消化　依照传代的方法用 0.25% 胰蛋白酶对处于对数生长期的单层细胞进行消化。收集消化细胞于离心管中,800~1 000r/min 离心 5min。

3. 稀释及分装　弃上清,加适量冻存液,吸管吹打、制悬,计数,调整细胞密度为 $(5\sim10) \times 10^6$ 个 /ml。每个冻存管分装细胞悬液 1~1.5ml,旋紧冻存管的管盖并封严,在冻存管上标明细胞的名称、冻存时间及操作者。

冻存:将冻存管置于如下条件下逐步加以冻存:4℃,30min → –20℃,30~60min → –80℃,过夜（16~18h）→液氮。

【实验结果】

1. 组织块法培养的细胞　培养 24h 后,倒置显微镜下可观察到少量形态不规则的细胞从心肌组织块边缘游离出来;48h 后,可见大量的细胞呈放射状排列于组织块周围,逐渐向外扩展连成一片。靠近组织块的细胞胞体较小且圆,距离组织块较远的区域可见多角形细胞,体积较大,还有些细胞的形态介于圆形与多角形之间。这些细胞彼此间排列紧密,细胞核较大,细胞质内含物少,透明度高。

2. 消化法培养的细胞　在倒置显微镜下观察,可见刚接种于培养瓶中的细胞均为圆形,悬浮于培养液中;接种 12h 后大部分细胞贴壁;24h 后细胞几乎全部贴壁,贴壁细胞伸出伪足,呈梭形、三角形等（图 9-2）;48h 后,心

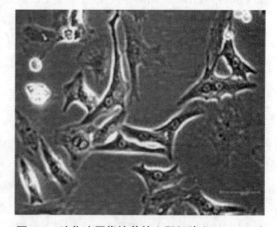

图 9-2　消化法原代培养的心肌细胞（24h,×200）

肌细胞伪足间形成连接,交织成网状。

3. 传代培养的细胞　贴壁生长的细胞,通常传代培养 2h 左右,细胞即能贴壁生长,2~4h 可形成单层。培养过程中,可通过 0.4% 锥虫蓝染色了解培养细胞中死细胞、活细胞的比例。悬浮型细胞传代后,一般 12h 后观察细胞是否被污染,细胞形态是否正常,细胞数量是否增加,如有必要可以锥虫蓝染色观察活细胞、死细胞比例。

【附】细胞培养的无菌操作要求

细胞培养是一种程序复杂、条件较多且要求严格的实验性工作。完善准备工作是决定细胞培养成功与否的首要条件,应给予足够重视,即便使用设备完善和条件优越的实验室,若实验者粗心大意,技术操作不规范,可能导致实验进展不顺。准备工作的内容包括器皿的清洗、干燥与消毒,培养液与其他试剂的配制、分装及灭菌,无菌室或超净台的清洁与消毒,培养箱及其他仪器的检查与调试等。特别要注意无菌操作,这是细胞体外培养成败的关键。

1. 器材和液体的准备　细胞培养用的玻璃器材,如:培养瓶、吸管等清洗干净后装在铝盒或铁筒中,120℃,2h 干烤灭菌后备用;手术器材、瓶塞、配制好的 PBS 液于灭菌锅 103.4kPa,20min 灭菌;培养液、小牛血清、消化液等用 G6 滤器负压抽滤后备用。

2. 无菌操作注意事项　操作前 20~30min 启动超净台吹风,认真洗手并用 75% 乙醇消毒。操作时严禁说话,用止血钳、镊子等器械拿瓶塞等无菌物品,严禁用手直接接触。培养瓶开瓶塞及开瓶后的操作必须在超净台内完成,开塞前乙醇消毒瓶口,开塞后和加塞前瓶口需酒精灯过火,操作完毕塞瓶塞后才可拿到超净台外。整个操作过程都应于酒精灯的周围进行,以保证工作区无菌清洁。

【分析思考】

1. 贴壁细胞和悬浮细胞在传代方法上有什么不同?

2. 为什么培养细胞长成致密单层后必须要进行传代培养?

3. 原代培养和传代培养有哪些区别?

4. 细胞培养过程中,培养液颜色为什么会变黄? 避免污染的关键环节有哪些?

5. 细胞冻存过程中加入 DMSO 与缓慢降温的原理是什么?

【实验报告】

完成细胞原代培养、传代培养与冻存的实验记录。

实验 10　细胞增殖检测(CCK8 法)

【目的要求】

掌握 CCK8 检测细胞增殖的原理和方法。

【实验原理】

细胞增殖是指细胞在周期调控因子作用下,通过 DNA 复制、RNA 转录和蛋白质合成等反应,完成细胞分裂的过程,是生物体的重要生命特征。增殖检测一般是分析分裂中的细胞数量的变化,进而反映细胞的生长状态及活性,目前广泛应用于肿瘤生物学、遗传学、分子生物学和药代动力学等领域。

目前细胞增殖的检测方法包括细胞数量检测(直接计数法)、DNA 合成检测(BrdU 和 EdU 检测)、细胞周期检测(流式细胞仪 PI 染色法)、代谢活性检测(MTT、CCK8 法等)、细胞

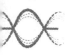

增殖相关抗原检测（如 Ki-67 蛋白检测）、ATP 浓度检测（荧光素酶催化反应）等，选择何种方法应该根据细胞类型和实验需求而定。

丝裂霉素 C 是从头状链霉菌培养液中分离提取的一种细胞周期非特异性药物，可通过与 DNA 分子的双螺旋形成交联，破坏 DNA 的结构和功能，进而抑制有丝分裂间期 DNA 的复制，对体外培养的细胞有毒性作用。

CCK8 全称 Cell Counting Kit-8 试剂，该试剂含有 WST-8，WST-8 的化学名称为 2-（2- 甲氧基 -4- 硝苯基）-3-（4- 硝苯基）-5-（2,4- 二磺基苯）-2H- 四唑单钠盐，在电子载体存在的情况下，WST-8 被细胞内脱氢酶氧化还原后生成水溶性的橙黄色甲臜染料，能够溶解在组织培养液中，生成的甲臜量与活细胞数量成正比。细胞增殖越多越快，则颜色越深；细胞毒性越大，则颜色越浅。对同样的细胞，颜色深浅和细胞数量呈线性关系，用酶标仪在 450nm 波长处测定 OD 值，可间接反映出细胞的数量，因此可利用这一特性直接进行细胞增殖和毒性分析，且此种方法操作简便、灵敏度高、细胞毒性小。

【实验用品】

（一）材料

人 U251 胶质瘤细胞。

（二）器材

CO_2 培养箱、倒置显微镜、荧光显微镜、离心机、酶标仪、酒精灯、细胞计数板、乳胶头吸管、培养瓶、离心管、96 孔细胞培养板、移液器及枪头。

（三）试剂

0.25% 胰蛋白酶、含有 10% 小牛血清的 DMEM/F12 培养液、PBS、丝裂霉素 C 溶液（基础培养液配制）、CCK8 试剂盒。

【实验步骤】

1. 制备细胞悬液　收集对数期 U251 细胞后离心，并使用新鲜配液重悬、计数，使细胞浓度为 $(2{\sim}3) \times 10^4$ 个 /ml。

2. 接种　将细胞悬液接种到 96 孔板中，每孔约 100μl。

3. 培养　将接种好细胞的 96 孔板放入 CO_2 培养箱（37℃）中，培养 24h。

4. 给药及分组　对照孔不处理，直接放入培养箱中过夜；实验孔吸出培养液，按照浓度梯度配制丝裂霉素 C 培养液（一般是 0、10、25、50、100mg/L），每孔加入 200μl，每个浓度设置 5 个复孔，并将 96 孔板放入 CO_2 培养箱培养过夜。

5. 加入 CCK8　每孔加入 10μl 的 CCK8 试剂，为避免因试剂沾在孔壁上导致误差，建议在加完试剂后轻轻敲击培养板以助混匀；或直接加入含 10%CCK8 的培养液，以换液的形式加入。并于培养箱中孵育 2h。

6. 测定 450nm 吸光度，以 OD 值为纵坐标，药物浓度为横坐标绘制曲线，根据下列公式进行计算并作图。

$$细胞存活率 =[(As{-}Ab)/(Ac{-}Ab)] \times 100\%$$
$$抑制率 =[(Ac{-}As)/(Ac{-}Ab)] \times 100\%$$

As：实验孔吸光度（含细胞、培养液、CCK-8 试剂和药物溶液）；

Ac：对照孔吸光度（含细胞、培养液、CCK-8 试剂，不含药物）；

Ab：空白孔吸光度（含培养液、CCK-8 试剂，不含细胞、药物）。

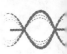

【分析思考】

1. 如何减少由于 CCK-8 试剂在枪头上或孔壁上的残留所带来的误差？

2. 在实验中 OD 值太高或太低，该如何解决？

3. 实验之前，是否需要先检测一下培养液和 CCK-8 是否会反应？

【实验报告】

分析不同浓度丝裂霉素 C 处理对 U251 胶质瘤细胞增殖的影响。

实验 11　细胞凋亡检测

【目的要求】

熟悉荧光染色的方法及光镜下凋亡细胞、坏死细胞和活细胞的鉴别。

【实验原理】

细胞凋亡（apoptosis），也称细胞程序性死亡，是指为维持内环境稳定，由基因控制的细胞自主有序的死亡过程。细胞凋亡是生物体中一种普遍存在的现象，胚胎形成、个体发育、衰老和损伤细胞的清除等都与细胞凋亡密切相关，此过程涉及一系列基因的激活、表达以及调控等的作用。

过氧化氢（H_2O_2）是一种强氧化剂，可以通过破坏正常线粒体功能和损伤 DNA 诱导氧化应激，导致活性氧含量增加，从而激活"内源性凋亡"或线粒体凋亡途径。细胞凋亡时，其细胞核染色质的 DNA 出现缺口甚至断裂，致使染色质凝聚、边缘化甚至呈现 DNA 碎片，利用与 DNA 结合的荧光染料染色后，在荧光显微镜下即可观察到上述变化。

正常细胞质膜的磷脂分布是不对称的，活细胞中磷脂酰丝氨酸（PS）位于细胞质膜的内表面。在细胞凋亡早期，PS 从细胞质膜的内表面翻转到细胞质膜的外表面。Annexin V 是一种对 PS 有高度亲和力的钙依赖性的磷脂结合蛋白。以标记荧光素 FITC 的 Annexin V 作为探针，利用流式细胞仪或荧光显微镜可检测细胞凋亡的发生。而坏死细胞的 PS 也会从细胞质膜的内表面翻转到细胞质膜的外表面，所以 Annexin V 无法区分坏死细胞和凋亡细胞。碘化丙啶（PI）是一种核酸染料，早期凋亡细胞和活细胞的细胞质膜仍然完整，PI 无法自由通过细胞质膜，所以无法标记凋亡细胞和活细胞，而 PI 却能够通过坏死细胞的细胞质膜与细胞内的 DNA 结合，区分坏死细胞和活细胞。所以 Annexin V 和 PI 同时使用，就可以区分活细胞、早期凋亡细胞、晚期凋亡细胞和坏死细胞。

【实验用品】

（一）材料

人神经胶质细胞瘤细胞（U251 细胞）。

（二）器材

CO_2 培养箱、超净工作台、倒置显微镜、荧光显微镜、移液器、小离心管、24 孔细胞培养板等。

（三）试剂

H_2O_2、PBS、Annexin V/PI 双染试剂盒（含 Binding Buffer、Annexin V-FITC 和 PI）、DMEM/F12 细胞培养液（含 10% 小牛血清）、75% 乙醇。

【实验步骤】

1. 培养细胞　将生长状态良好的 U251 细胞传代接种于 24 孔板，37℃的 CO_2 培养

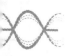
养 24h。

2. 诱导凋亡　从细胞培养板中移去培养液,加 2ml PBS,洗涤细胞 1 次。再加入含有不同浓度梯度的 H_2O_2(使用无血清 DMEM 培养液配制浓度分别为 0、50μmol/L、100μmol/L、150μmol/L、200μmol/L 和 400μmol/L 的 H_2O_2),每孔加 2ml,至少设计 3 个复孔,室温放置 5min。

3. 染色及分组　阴性对照组:不添加染色剂,直接在荧光显微镜下观察;实验组:吸出 H_2O_2 处理过的细胞中的液体,用 PBS 洗 1 次,每孔加入 Binding Buffer100μl 和 Annexin V-FITC 1μl,室温避光孵育 30min 后,每孔加入 PI 1μl,避光反应 5min 后立即在荧光显微镜下拍照并计数计算凋亡率;阳性对照组:使用 75% 乙醇处理正常细胞 5min,使细胞质膜完全破坏,将乙醇吸出后,按实验组的方法染色、拍照、计数及计算凋亡率。

【实验结果】

在荧光显微镜下观察:绿色荧光为 AnnexinV-FITC 染色阳性细胞,红色荧光为 PI 染色阳性细胞。仅被绿色荧光染色的为早期凋亡细胞,被绿色荧光和红色荧光双染的是晚期凋亡和坏死细胞,未被荧光染色的为正常细胞(见文末插图 11-1)。

【分析思考】

1. 简述细胞凋亡与细胞坏死的区别与联系。

2. AnnexinV-FITC/PI 双染检测细胞凋亡的原理是什么?

3. H_2O_2 诱导细胞凋亡的原理是什么?

【实验报告】

观察并记录凋亡细胞的形态特征。

实验 12　人类性染色质检测

【目的要求】

1. 熟悉性染色质标本的制备方法及临床意义。

2. 掌握性染色质的形态特征及识别方法。

【实验原理】

性染色质指人的体细胞间期细胞核中的 X 染色质和 Y 染色质。

X 染色质(X chromatin)是 Barr 和 Bertram 于 1949 年在雌猫神经细胞核中发现的,也称为 Barr 小体或 X 小体,雄猫神经细胞核中则没有这种结构。进一步研究发现,除雌猫以外,其他雌性哺乳动物及正常女性间期细胞核中均存在这种结构。

赖昂假说对此的解释是:正常女性或其他雌性哺乳动物体细胞中的 2 条 X 染色体,间期只有一条有活性,另一条失活呈异固缩状态,形成 X 染色质。正常男性体细胞中只有 1 条 X 染色体,不失活,故见不到 X 染色质。X 染色体数目异常的患者,体细胞中只有 1 条 X 染色体有活性,其余的 X 染色体均失活形成 X 染色质,例如,核型为 47,XXX 和 48,XXXY 的个体均有 2 个 X 染色质;而核型为 48,XXXX 的个体则有 3 个 X 染色质。对任何个体而言,体细胞中的 X 染色质数等于 X 染色体数减 1。

男性体细胞中期分裂象用荧光染料染色,可见 Y 染色体长臂远端(q12)发出强荧光;如用荧光染料对男性间期细胞染色,则细胞核内可看到一个直径约 0.3μm 的强荧光小体,这说明此强荧光小体与 Y 染色体长臂远端的强荧光区是一致的,此荧光小体称为 Y 染色质(Y chromatin)或 Y 小体(Y body)。男性间期细胞核的强荧光小体及 Y 染色体上的强荧光区是由 Y 染色体长臂远端的结构决定的,即此结构对荧光染料有较强的亲合力。

因此,性染色质的检测是判断性别的简便方法,也是临床上性染色体病诊断和产前诊断的辅助手段。理论上,正常女性体细胞中均应见到 1 个 X 染色质,正常男性体细胞中均应见到 1 个 Y 染色质,但由于受到个体的生理状态、染色方法、X 染色质或 Y 染色质存在位置及其他未知因素的影响,故 X 染色质及 Y 染色质的阳性率较低。

【实验用品】

（一）材料

正常男性和正常女性口腔黏膜细胞、毛囊细胞,正常男性外周血白细胞。

（二）器材

载玻片、盖玻片、牙签、刀片、染色缸、酒精灯、显微镜、荧光显微镜、擦镜纸。

（三）试剂

5mol/L HCl 溶液、0.5% 盐酸喹吖因溶液、0.2% 甲苯胺蓝液、Giemsa 染液、Carnoy 固定液、95% 乙醇、40% 醋酸、爽口液、硫堇染液、指甲油、蒸馏水。

【实验步骤】

（一）X 染色质

1. 取材、制片和固定

（1）口腔黏膜细胞:女性受试者用爽口液漱口,清净口腔,用牙签钝端在口腔颊部黏膜表面刮取较深层的黏膜细胞,刮取时需稍用力,也可用另一只手的示指在面颊外顶住稍稍加压。将细胞均匀涂在载玻片上,自然干燥。为保证获得较深层的上皮细胞,可弃去第一次刮取物。将涂片放入 Carnoy 固定液中,固定 15min,自然干燥。

（2）毛囊细胞:女性受试者拔下 2~3 根头发,将根部带有完整毛囊组织的部分置于载玻片中央,加 1 滴 40% 醋酸处理 10min,将毛囊软化,用刀片轻轻将毛囊组织刮在载玻片中央并用牙签均匀涂布,在酒精灯上远火微烤,使其干燥,加 1 滴 Carnoy 固定液,固定 15min。

2. 水解　将固定后自然干燥的载玻片浸入 5mol/L HCl 溶液中水解 10min,自来水冲洗,晾干。

3. 染色　载玻片上滴数滴硫堇染液(或 0.2% 甲苯胺蓝染液或 Giemsa 染液),染色 5~10min,自来水冲洗,晾干。

4. 镜检　低倍镜下,可见细胞核为圆形或卵圆形,染成紫蓝色,细胞质不着色。寻找铺展较好的细胞移置视野中央,换油镜,选择典型的可计数细胞进一步观察。

可计数细胞的判断标准是:细胞核较大,轮廓清楚、核膜完整无缺损,染色深浅适中,核内染色质呈细丝状或均匀的细颗粒状、细胞核内无其他块状颗粒,核膜周围无细菌污染。可计数细胞核内,X 染色质的特征是:位于核膜内缘、轮廓清晰,结构致密而染色较深,呈圆形、卵圆形、三角形或馒头状等,直径 1~1.5μm(图 12-1A)。观察 100 个细胞,统计 X 染色质的阳性率。X 染色质的出现率一般为 20%~30%。

（二）Y 染色质

1. 取材、制片和固定

（1）口腔黏膜细胞(男性):同前。

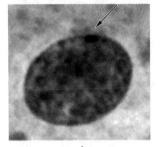

A

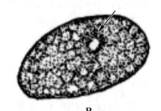

B

图 12-1　X 染色质和 Y 染色质

A. X 染色质;B. Y 染色质。

（2）毛囊细胞（男性）：同前。

（3）外周血白细胞（男性）：按血涂片的制备方法（实验二）制成血涂片，95%乙醇固定15min，晾干。此标本可显示淋巴细胞、粒细胞和单核细胞的Y染色质。

2. 染色　将标本片浸入0.5%氮芥喹吖因溶液的染色缸中染色6min。

3. 分色　取出标本片，放入蒸馏水中漂洗10min，洗去染液、分色。

4. 封片　从蒸馏水中取出标本片，立即加1~2滴蒸馏水在标本上，然后盖上盖玻片。为避免干燥、水分蒸发，可在盖玻片周围用指甲油密封。

5. 镜检　标本静置片刻，放入荧光显微镜下观察。低倍镜下，可见许多黄色的细胞核。换高倍镜或油镜进一步观察。细胞核内呈现的较强荧光亮点即为Y染色质（Y小体），此荧光亮点闪烁如星，位于核的中部或边缘，直径0.25~0.3μm（见图12-1B）。

观察100个细胞，统计Y染色质的阳性率。计数的细胞必须核膜完整无缺，核质染色均匀，清晰可见，细胞核周围无细菌和其他污染物质干扰。Y染色质的阳性率个体差异较大，男性口腔黏膜细胞的阳性率一般为20%~30%，男性白细胞的阳性率为10%~30%，但二者均可高达70%。

【分析思考】
1. X染色质和Y染色质标本制备过程应注意哪些问题？
2. X染色质与X染色体、Y染色质和Y染色体是何关系？
3. 性染色质的检测在临床上有何应用价值？

【实验报告】
绘图：X染色质和Y染色质。

实验13　小鼠骨髓细胞染色体标本的制备

【目的要求】
1. 掌握动物骨髓细胞染色体标本制备的方法。
2. 熟悉小鼠骨髓细胞染色体的形态和数目。

【实验原理】
染色体是染色质的高度凝集状态，观察典型染色体的形态，必须获得有丝分裂中期分裂象。骨髓细胞始终保持较强的分裂活性，且细胞数量较多，直接利用骨髓细胞制备染色体标本比利用其他组织可获得更多的分裂象。该方法简便易行，不需特殊的设备和无菌操作。因此，骨髓细胞是制作动物细胞染色体标本的理想材料。动物活体内注射秋水仙碱，可抑制细胞分裂时的纺锤体形成，使处于增殖状态的骨髓细胞停止在中期；中期分裂细胞，经低渗处理，可使细胞质膜胀破、染色体分散；固定剂处理可使染色体结构清晰。

【实验用品】
（一）材料
小鼠。

（二）器材
解剖盘、解剖剪、解剖针、镊子、吸管、刻度离心管、培养皿、5ml注射器、1ml注射器、5号针头、6号针头、离心机、普通天平、试管架、冷藏载玻片、记号笔、酒精灯、恒温水浴箱、载玻片、吸水纸、显微镜、香柏油（或液体石蜡）、无水乙醇（或乙醚乙醇混合液）、擦镜纸。

（三）试剂

10%Giemsa 染液、Carnoy 固定液、0.01% 秋水仙碱、0.075mol/L KCl 低渗液、0.9%NaCl 溶液。

【实验步骤】

1. 动物预处理　取小鼠 1 只，在天平上称重，按 1~2μg/g（体重）的注射剂量，实验前 3~4h，用 1ml 注射器（5 号针头）给小鼠腹腔注射秋水仙碱，即每 10g 体重注射 0.01% 秋水仙碱 0.1~0.2ml。

2. 取材　用颈椎脱臼法处死小鼠，立即用剪刀和镊子剪开后肢大腿上的皮肤和肌肉，暴露出股骨及其两端的关节，完整取出两根股骨，剔除骨上残余的肌肉和肌腱。

3. 收集细胞　剪去股骨两端少量骨质，暴露出骨髓腔，用解剖针将两端穿透；用镊子夹住股骨中部，用 5ml 注射器（6 号针头）抽取 4ml 0.9%NaCl 溶液，将针头插入骨髓腔，冲洗腔内的骨髓细胞；将冲洗液直接收集到刻度离心管中，反复数次，直到股骨发白为止。

用吸管反复吸打离心管内的收集液，待其中组织块自然沉降后，吸出上层细胞悬液至另一离心管中，以 1 000r/min，离心 8~10min，吸弃上清液。

4. 低渗　在含骨髓细胞的离心管中加入 37℃ 预温的 0.075mol/L KCl 低渗液 5ml，用吸管轻轻吹打混匀，置 37℃ 的恒温水浴箱中，低渗处理 30min。

5. 预固定　在终止低渗前 1~2min，加入新配的 Carnoy 固定液 0.5~1ml 打匀，预固定。预固定 5min 后，1 000r/min 离心 8~10min，吸弃上清液。

6. 固定　用吸管沿离心管壁缓慢加入 Carnoy 固定液 5~6ml，轻轻将沉淀冲散打匀，室温下静置固定 15~20min。1 000r/min 离心 8~10min，吸弃上清液。重复此固定和离心过程 1 次。

7. 制备细胞悬液　视离心管中沉淀物量的多少加入适量新配制的 Carnoy 固定液（约 0.3ml），用吸管缓慢打匀成细胞悬液。

8. 制片　从冰箱中取出冰冷的载玻片，平铺于滴片架上用吸管吸取少许细胞悬液，使吸管口距离载玻片 20~30cm，将细胞悬液滴于载玻片上（每片 2~3 滴，不要重叠），立即对准所滴液体微微吹气，使细胞悬液在玻片上散开，再将载玻片掠过酒精灯几次（标本面朝上，载玻片距离火焰不要太近），有利于染色体更好地分散和展开。玻片置空气中自然干燥后，用记号笔在标本面做上标记。

9. 染色　将标本片平排于染色架上，标本面向上，用吸管吸取 10%Giemsa 染液滴于标本片上，染色 15~20min，流水冲去染液，自然晾干。

10. 镜检　低倍镜下可见许多大小不等、染成紫红色的间期细胞核和分散其间的中期分裂象，选择染色体形态好、分散均匀的中期分裂象，换用油镜观察。

（1）染色体计数：根据分裂象中染色体的自然分布状态，将其中的染色体分成几个区域，分别计数各区的染色体数，然后将各区的染色体数相加即为该细胞的染色体总数。小鼠体细胞染色体数为 2n=40，雄鼠为 19 对常染色体和 X、Y 性染色体，雌鼠为 19 对常染色体和 X、X 性染色体。

（2）染色体形态观察：小鼠染色体全部为端着丝粒染色体，呈 U 形。X 染色体大小介于 5~6 号染色体之间，Y 染色体最小（图 13-1）。

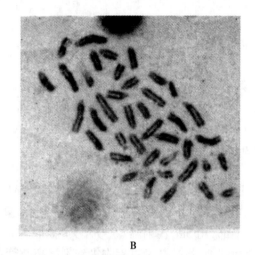

图 13-1 小鼠骨髓细胞中期染色体

A. 模式图;B. 显微结构图。

【分析思考】

1. 本实验中秋水仙碱和低渗液各起什么作用?

2. 低渗时间过长或过短对染色体会有何影响?

【实验报告】

绘小鼠骨髓细胞中期分裂象。

实验 14 人类 G 显带染色体核型分析

【目的要求】

1. 初步掌握胰蛋白酶法人类染色体 G 显带技术。

2. 初步掌握 G 显带染色体核型分析方法。

3. 了解人类 G 显带染色体带纹主要特征。

【实验原理】

染色体标本经物理、化学因素处理,并用特定染料分化染色,每条染色体上呈现的明暗相间或深浅不同横纹,称为染色体带纹,简称为带。显示染色体带的实验方法称为显带技术(banding technique)。染色体带的数目、部位、宽窄和着色深浅均具有相对稳定性,每号染色体都有固定的带纹构成,称为带型。这说明染色体本身存在能显带的结构。

显带技术不同,染色体上显示出的带纹也不同。染色体显带技术包括 G 显带、Q 显带、R 显带、C 显带等。G 显带(G banding)技术简便易行,所显示的染色体带纹清晰、普通显微镜下可以分辨,标本可长期保存,因此被广泛应用。

同源染色体的带型基本稳定,不同对染色体带型不同,因此,通过 G 显带染色体的核型分析,不仅可准确识别每一号染色体,而且可发现染色体上细微的结构变化,是早期基因定位、区域制图及染色体病诊断的一项常用技术。

【实验用品】

(一)材料

未染色的人类染色体标本片(白片)、G 显带染色体核型照片。

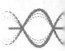

（二）器材

恒温水浴箱、烤箱、立式染缸、直头小吸管、橡皮吸头、剪刀、镊子、胶水、牙签、显微镜、香柏油（或液体石蜡）、无水乙醇（或乙醚乙醇混合液）、擦镜纸。

（三）试剂

0.1% 胰蛋白酶溶液、3%Tris、0.4% 酚红、3%Giemsa 染液、蒸馏水。

【实验步骤】

（一）显带机制简介

染色体带型主要取决于 DNA、蛋白质及染料三者的相互作用，即特定碱基组成的 DNA 与 DNA 结合蛋白形成的特定结构对染料分子的作用。Summer（1974）的实验表明，DNA 分子的螺旋与折叠、非组蛋白的分布，在染色体上呈区域性差异；这些差异导致二硫键与硫氢键分布不同，许多二硫键交联的区域易与染料结合呈深染区，而缺乏二硫键、多硫氢键，不易与染料结合的区域则浅染。

Lee 等认为，与 DNA 分子结合疏松的组蛋白，易被胰蛋白酶分解，该染色体区段显示浅染带；反之，与 DNA 分子牢固结合的组蛋白，不易被胰蛋白酶分解，则该染色体区段显示深染带。一般认为，易着色的阳性带是富含 A-T 的染色体节段；相反，富含 G-C 的节段不易着色。尽管如此，总的来说，染色体显带的机制尚不清楚。

（二）胰蛋白酶法 G 显带技术简介

1. 标本选择　长度适中、分散好、重叠少、姐妹染色单体适度分开的染色体标本片适于 G 显带。

2. 烤片　片龄 3~7d 的染色体标本片，放入 60℃烤箱中烤片 2~12h，自然冷却至室温。

3. 胰蛋白酶预温　将盛有 0.1% 胰蛋白酶溶液的染色缸放入 37℃恒温水浴箱内预温，在染色缸内加入 0.4% 酚红 1 滴，再用 3%Tris 调节 pH 至 7.0。

4. 显带　当胰蛋白酶溶液温度达 37℃时，将标本片浸入胰蛋白酶溶液中，轻轻连续摆动（消化），为确定最佳消化时间，第 1 张标本片分成 3 段进行预消化，例如，第 1 段消化 15s，第 2 段消化 13s，第 3 段消化 10s。

5. 染色　取出标本片，立即用蒸馏水漂洗，去除标本片上残留的胰蛋白酶溶液；将标本片放入 37℃预温、含 3%Giemsa 染液的染色缸中染色 5~8min；自来水轻轻冲洗标本片上染液，晾干。

6. 镜检　先在低倍镜下寻找分裂象，然后在油镜下观察，根据染色体显带及染色情况，调整下一张标本片的消化及染色时间，直至摸索到合适的消化及染色时间。如果标本上染色体呈蓝紫色，说明胰蛋白酶的作用时间不够；如果染色体呈桃红色，则比较合适。

（三）影响 G 显带效果的主要因素

1. 标本片的质量　标本片上染色体相对较长，早中期的分裂象最理想，分裂象较多，多分散均匀。

2. 胰蛋白酶溶液的浓度和温度　浓度高时，消化所需时间变短，且易消化过头。因此，胰蛋白酶浓度不宜过高，通常消化时间不宜少于 10s。胰蛋白酶最适作用温度为 37℃，如温度较低，则消化所需时间延长。

3. 片龄　标本片保存时间越长，染色体对胰蛋白酶处理的抵抗性越大。片龄超过 20d 的标本片，显带时染色体往往呈斑点状，而不显示带纹。

4. 染液　染液须现用现配，保存时间不应超过 48h。

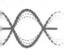

（四）G 显带染色体核型分析

1. 镜下核型分析　低倍镜下,可见许多转化或未转化的圆形淋巴细胞,染色体被染成紫色或紫红色。选择染色体形态和分散良好的中期分裂象,移到视野中心,换高倍镜观察;高倍镜下观察分裂象中染色体的显带情况,选择染色体分散良好、互不重叠、长度适中、显带好(深浅带清楚,边缘清晰)、染色良好的分裂象换油镜观察。

油镜下先进行染色体计数,至少要计数 10 个分裂象的染色体数;然后观察染色体的形态、着丝粒位置;根据染色体的带纹特征,仔细辨认每条染色体,判断被检者细胞的染色体有无异常。对于初学者,在油镜下区别各号染色体较难,可先试着用铅笔画出镜下所见的显带染色体草图,然后根据染色体的带纹特点,在画出的染色体旁标上号数。

为判断性别,要着重掌握 21 号、22 号及 X、Y 染色体的带纹特征。如观察到最小的近端着丝粒染色体(G 组)是 5 条,并且能确认有一个 Y 染色体和一个 X 染色体,则可判断为正常男性;如果 G 组染色体数目是 4 条,并且确认有 2 条 X 染色体,则判断为正常女性。图 14-1 是人显带染色体标准带型图,由于受实验条件及其他因素的影响,通常 G 显带技术显示的带纹数少于标准带型。

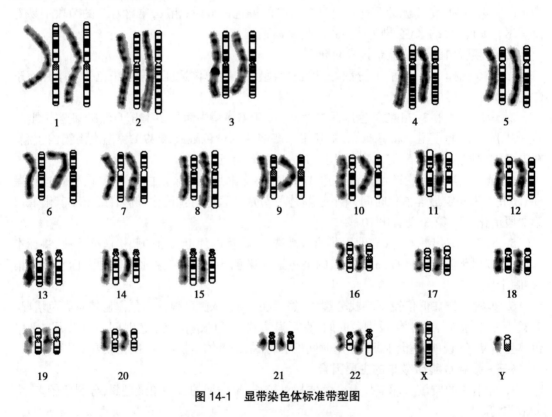

图 14-1　显带染色体标准带型图

在实际工作中,人们归纳、总结了各号染色体 G 带带纹的主要特征,并编成 G 带歌诀;在理解的基础上熟记 G 带歌诀,有助于掌握 G 带染色体的带纹特征,从而识别各号染色体。

【附】G 带歌诀

一秃二蛇三蝶飘,四像鞭炮五黑腰。六号短空小白脸,七盖八下九苗条。

十号 q 三近带好,十一低来十二高。十三十四十五号,3 个长臂一二一。

十六长臂缢痕大,十七长远戴脚镣。十八白头肚子大,十九中间一黑腰。

二十头重脚底轻,二十一像葫芦瓢。二十二一点 Y 黑腰,Xpq 一肩挑。

2. 核型照片分析　G 显带核型照片分析的方法与非显带染色体核型照片分析相似,先根据各组染色体的结构特征,依次找出 A、B、D、E、F、G 组,剩余的为 C 组,在每条染色体旁用铅笔标出组号;然后根据 G 带的带纹特征,进一步标出染色体序号;用剪刀将每条染色体连同组号、序号剪下;按照染色体序号依次配对排列,此时如发现识别有误,可进行调整;最后,将染色体组号、序号剪去,将各号染色体排在染色体核型分析表的相应位置上,用胶水贴牢。粘贴时,应使染色体的短臂向上、长臂向下,并使着丝粒在一条直线上(图 14-2、图 14-3)。剪贴过程要细心,防止丢失染色体。正确剪贴后,书写被检细胞的核型。

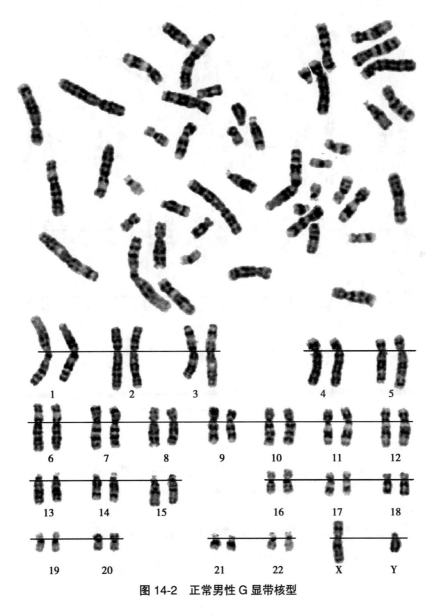

图 14-2　正常男性 G 显带核型

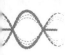

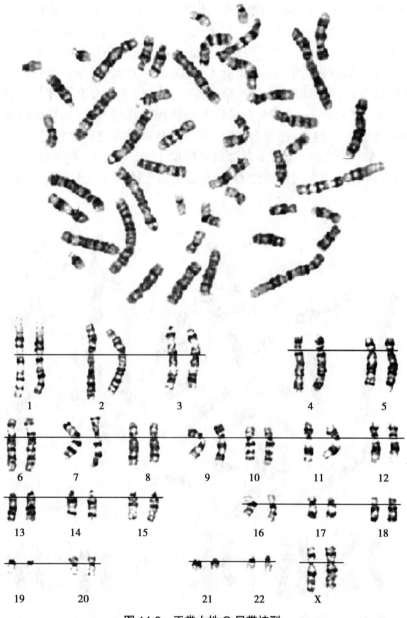

图 14-3 正常女性 G 显带核型

【分析思考】

1. 要制备良好的 G 带染色体标本,实验操作时应注意哪些问题?

2. 试述正常人类染色体 G 带带纹主要特征。

【实验报告】

正常男性 G 显带染色体核型剪贴分析(图 14-4,见文末插图 14-5)。

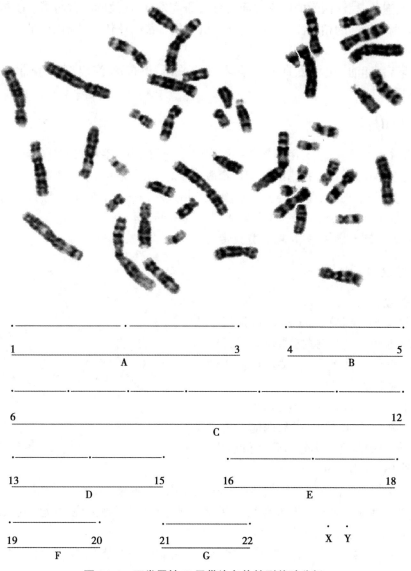

图 14-4　正常男性 G 显带染色体核型剪贴分析

实验 15　人类皮肤纹理分析

【目的要求】

1. 掌握皮肤纹理的分析方法及正常人的皮肤纹理特点。
2. 熟悉皮肤纹理异常与遗传病的关系。

【实验原理】

皮肤纹理（dermatoglyph），简称皮纹，是指手足掌面呈现的纹理。在胚胎发育过程中，真皮乳头向表皮突出形成的乳头线，在皮肤表面呈现出凸起的条纹，称为嵴纹（ridge），嵴纹之间的凹陷称为沟纹（furrow），嵴纹和沟纹相间排列构成皮纹。

人体的皮纹属于多基因遗传，是在遗传因素和环境因素的相互作用下形成的，具有高度稳定性，出生前就已定型，终身不变；同时具有个体特异性。皮纹学的知识和技术，已广泛应用于人类学、遗传学、法医学的研究方面;另外,研究发现,皮纹的异常与某些遗传性疾病,尤其是染色体病有较高的相关性,因此,皮纹分析可用于某些遗传病的辅助诊断。

【实验用品】

器材:印台、印油、放大镜、直尺、量角器、8 开白纸、擦布、洗涤剂、宽窄胶带、铅笔。

【实验步骤】

一、拓印皮纹

受检者洗净双手并擦干,用铅笔在一张白纸上均匀涂黑,手指末节及侧面由一侧向另一侧滚转重复涂黑,然后把手指指纹拓印在窄胶带上,依次印取 10 个手指的指纹,之后把印上指纹的胶带剪下粘贴在实验报告上。若印取的指纹不清晰,需重印。最后,从拇指侧开始,依次标上指号 1、2、3、4、5,记录被取指纹者姓名、拓印时间。

掌纹也需要同上操作,只是粘在宽胶带上。

二、皮纹分析

(一) 指纹

1. 指纹类型　指纹(finger print)是指手指末节掌面的皮肤纹理,依据指端外侧三叉点的有无和数目分为 3 种类型,三叉点是指 3 种不同走向纹线的汇聚点(图 15-1)。

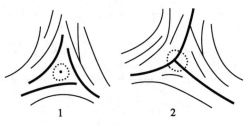

图 15-1　三叉点

(1) 弓形纹(arch,A):弓形纹的嵴纹从一侧走向另一侧,中间隆起如弓形,两侧均无三叉点。根据弓形纹的曲度大小分为简弓和帐弓(隆起度大)(图 15-2A、图 15-2B)。

(2) 箕形纹(loop,L):箕形纹的嵴纹从一侧发出,走向对侧指端,再折返回到同侧,形状似簸箕。箕口朝向尺侧者称为尺箕或正箕,箕口朝向桡侧者称为桡箕或反箕(图 15-2C、图 15-2D)。箕口的对侧有 1 个三叉点。

在正常人,桡箕少见,而第 4 指桡箕罕见。若见到较多的桡箕,特别是位于第 4、5 指时,则提示可能存在遗传学异常。

(3) 斗形纹(whorl,W):斗形纹的两侧各有 1 个三叉点,根据嵴纹的形状,斗形纹分为 3 种亚型(见图 15-2E、图 15-2F、图 15-2G):纹线呈同心圆形者称环形斗(circular whorl),纹线呈螺旋形者称螺形斗(spiral whorl),由 2 个箕形纹的箕头相互绞合组成的斗称双箕斗(double whorl)或绞形斗(wring whorl)。

各型指纹的分布及频率因人种而异,东方人多尺箕和斗形纹,弓形纹和桡箕少见;另外,还存在性别差异,与男性相比,女性弓形纹多,而斗形纹略少。

2. 指嵴纹计数

(1) 指嵴纹数:从箕形纹或斗形纹的纹心(core)向一侧或两侧三叉点连线,线段经过的嵴纹条数称为指嵴纹数(finger ridge count,FRC)。弓形纹无三叉点,指嵴纹数为 0;箕形纹一侧有三叉点,有 1 个指嵴纹数(图 15-3A);斗形纹两侧均有三叉点,有 2 个指嵴纹数,但只计指嵴纹数大者(图 15-3B)。双箕斗有 2 个纹心,自每一纹心向对侧三叉点连线,可得 2 个指嵴纹数;两纹心连线可得第 3 个指嵴纹数;三者相加除以 2,即得该双箕斗的指嵴纹

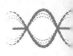

数（图 15-3C）。

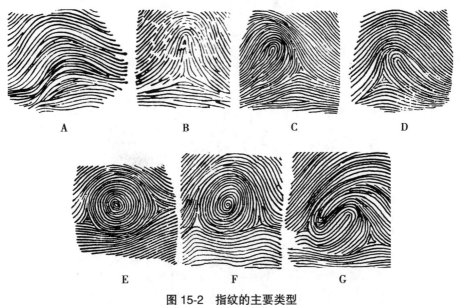

图 15-2　指纹的主要类型
A. 简弓；B. 帐弓；C. 尺箕；D. 桡箕；E. 环形斗；F. 螺形斗；G. 绞形斗（双箕斗）。

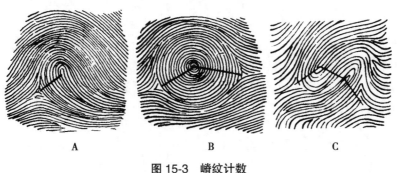

图 15-3　嵴纹计数
A. 箕形纹；B. 环形斗；C. 双箕斗。

　　（2）总指嵴纹数：将左右手 10 个手指的指嵴纹数相加为总指嵴纹数（total finger ridge count, TFRC）。国人斗形纹较多，故 TFRC 较高，汉族男性平均为 148.80，汉族女性平均为 138.46；欧美人斗形纹较少，故 TFRC 较低；另外，研究表明，性染色体病患者，随 X 染色体数目增多，TFRC 有递减的趋势。

　　（二）掌纹

　　手掌的皮肤纹理称掌纹（palmar print），掌纹主要包括以下类型（图 15-4）：

　　1. 真实花纹　大鱼际区（Th）、小鱼际区（Ty）及 5 个手指根部的 4 个指间区（I_1～I_4）均可出现类似指纹的弓形纹、箕形纹和斗形纹，其中箕形纹和斗形纹称为真实花纹。

　　2. 指三叉点与 a-b 嵴纹数　2~5 指根部各有 1 个三叉点，称为指三叉点，分别用 a、b、c、d 表示；a、b、c、d 发出的主要掌纹线分别称为 A 线、B 线、C 线和 D 线。在掌纹分析中，通常计数 a-b 嵴纹数，即 a、b 间连线，计数连线上的嵴纹数（起止点嵴纹不计），左手和右手 a-b 嵴纹数分别记录。国人的 a-b 嵴纹数为 40±1，低于欧美人；Turner 综合征患者 a-b 嵴纹数明显

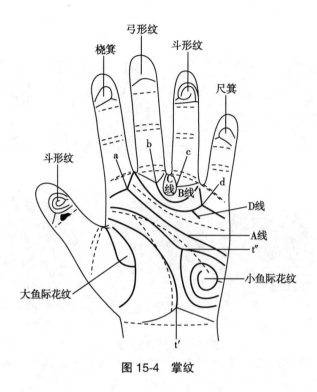

图 15-4 掌纹

增高。

3. 轴三叉点（atd 角） 轴三叉点位于大、小鱼际区之间的底端、手掌基部的正中附近，以 t 表示，也称 t 三叉点。t 三叉点的位置变化对某些染色体病的诊断具有重要意义，唐氏综合征等染色体病患者的 t 三叉点的位置往往偏高，甚至可达掌心。t 三叉点位置的定量描述方法有 atd 角和 t 距比两种（图 15-5）。

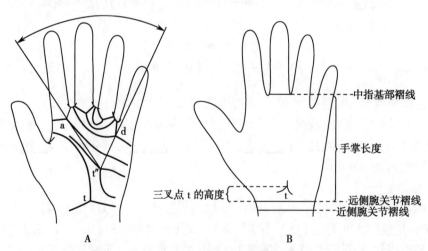

图 15-5 t 三叉点的定量描述

A. ∠atd 测量（本例为∠at″d）；B. t 距比测量。

（1）atd 角：分别连接三叉点 a、t 和 d，两线的夹角称为 atd 角（见图 15-5A）。国人的 atd 角平均值为 41°。atd 角越大，说明 t 三叉点越接近掌心；t 三叉点近掌心者称为 t″，介于 t 与 t″

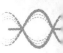

之间者称 t′。唐氏综合征患者的 at′d 角或 at″d 角平均值大于 64°（注意：无论正常人，还是染色体病患者，儿童期 atd 角均较成年期大）。

（2）t 距比：t 三叉点至远侧腕关节褶线的距离（三叉点 t 的高度）占手掌长度（远侧腕关节褶线至中指基部褶线的距离）的百分比称 t 距比（见图 15-5B）。t 距比通常小于 14.9%，t′ 距比为 15%~39.9%，而 t″ 距比则达 40%。

（三）褶纹

褶纹位于手指和手掌的屈面，由于关节的屈伸而形成。实际上，褶纹不属于皮肤纹理，但由于某些染色体病患者存在褶纹异常，故也将其列入皮纹介绍。

1. 指褶纹　正常人拇指有 1 条指褶纹，其余 4 指均有 2 条指褶纹，但唐氏综合征和 18 三体综合征患者第 5 指可只有 1 条指褶纹。

2. 掌褶纹　大多数正常人（约 90%）的手掌中通常有 3 条大的褶纹，分别是远侧横褶纹、近侧横褶纹和大鱼际褶纹（图 15-6），少数人呈变异型（图 15-7）。变异型中，4.2% 的个体为通贯掌或称猿线，即远侧和近侧横褶纹连接成单一的褶线，横贯全掌；5.8% 的个体为类似通贯掌，类似通贯掌又细分为 3 种类型：①变异Ⅰ型：远侧和近侧横褶纹借一条短褶纹彼此相连，横贯全掌，此型也称为桥贯掌；②变异Ⅱ型：一横褶纹通贯全掌，其上下有分支状小褶纹，此型也称为叉贯掌；③悉尼掌：远侧横褶纹和大鱼际褶纹与大多数正常人相同，而近侧横褶纹通贯全掌。此型常见于澳大利亚的悉尼人。智力低下的染色体病患者，通贯掌出现率较高；悉尼掌在白血病和先天愚型患者中出现率较高。

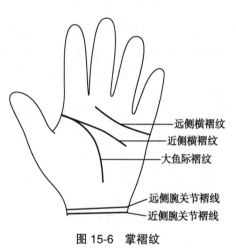

图 15-6　掌褶纹

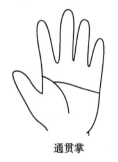
通贯掌

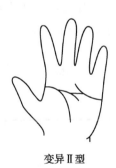
变异Ⅰ型　变异Ⅱ型

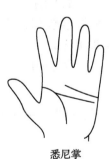
悉尼掌

图 15-7　变异型掌褶纹

（四）足纹

像手指和手掌一样，在足趾和足掌上也有相应的皮肤纹理，目前研究得较多、意义较大的是趾球区纹，它分为 7 种类型：①远侧箕形纹；②胫侧箕形纹；③腓侧箕形纹；④胫侧弓形纹；⑤腓侧弓形纹；⑥近侧弓形纹；⑦斗形纹。在 7 种足纹中，以胫侧弓形纹最为重要，其弓凹朝向胫侧，无三叉点；弓形弯度较小，近似平行；纹理密度小。此型在正常人中仅占 0.5%，但唐氏综合征患者的出现率可高达约 72%，该纹型是染色体病临床诊断的重要辅助指标。

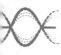

三、皮纹分析的临床意义

皮纹变化与某些遗传病,特别是染色体病有一定相关性,但其变化不是特异的,故只能作为疾病诊断的旁证或初筛,不能仅以此作为诊断依据,染色体核型分析是染色体病的确诊依据。

（一）染色体病

1. 唐氏综合征　患者指纹的斗形纹减少,箕形纹增多,特别是尺箕比例高,TFRC 较少,小指常单一指褶线,约 50% 患者出现通贯手,atd 角大于 60°,70% 以上患者有趾球区胫侧弓形纹。

2. 18 三体综合征　患者指纹的弓形纹比例增高,80% 患者有 7 个以上弓形纹（正常人出现 7 个以上弓形纹的概率仅 1%）,故 TFRC 值低;通贯手多见;约 25% 患者为 t″,约 40% 患者小指单一指褶线。

3. 13 三体综合征　桡箕和弓形纹显著增高,TFRC 低;50% 患者双手通贯手;轴三叉远移,约 81% 患者为 t″,趾球区腓侧弓形纹占 42%。

4. Turner 综合征　患者 TFRC 明显增加,atd 角增大,通贯手较多见,趾可见大斗形纹和远箕。

5. Klinefelter 综合征　弓形纹增多,TFRC 降低。

（二）双生子类型的判定

皮纹主要由遗传决定,同卵双生子的遗传基础相同,因此,同卵双生子的皮纹相似性必定很高;将皮纹分析与其他方法结合,区分同卵双生与异卵双生,可提高判定的准确率。

（三）个体识别

皮纹有个体特异性,且终生不变,可用做个体识别。

【分析思考】

1. 分析自己的指纹类型及嵴纹数、atd 角度及掌褶纹类型。
2. 哪些皮纹异常与染色体病相关联?

【实验报告】

填表:将自己的皮纹分析结果填入皮纹分析表。

附表:皮纹分析表

姓名			性别		年龄		民族		
手别			**左手**				**右手**		
		指别	1	2	3	4	5	1	2	3	4	5
指纹		指纹类型										
		指嵴纹数										
		总嵴纹数										
掌纹	真实花纹	区域										
		纹型										
	atd 角											
	掌长											

续表

手别		左手	右手
掌纹	t 距		
	t 距比（%）		
	a-b 嵴纹数		
褶纹	指褶纹		
	掌褶纹（正常型或变异型）		

实验 16　人类单基因遗传的群体分析

【目的要求】

1. 掌握 Hardy-Weinberg 定律在单基因遗传性状及单基因遗传病分析中的应用。

2. 熟悉遗传性状的调查分析方法；熟悉 PTC 尝味能力的检测方法，加深对单基因遗传规律的理解。

3. 了解人类某些遗传性状的遗传规律。

【实验用品】

吸管、梯度 PTC 溶液、蒸馏水。

【实验原理】

1. 苯硫脲（phenyl-thio-carbamide，PTC），白色结晶状，因含硫代酰胺基团而有苦涩味；PTC 对人无毒，亦无副作用。人类能否尝出 PTC 的苦涩味是由其基因决定的，呈不完全显性遗传：纯合尝味者的基因型为 TT，可尝出 PTC 的浓度为 1/768 000~1/614 400 000；味盲的基因型为 tt，PTC 的浓度≥1/24 000 方可尝出，有的味盲者甚至连 PTC 结晶粉末的苦涩味也尝不出；杂合子的基因型为 Tt，尝味能力介于纯合尝味者与味盲者之间，尝味等级为 1/48 000~1/384 000（表 16-1）。澳大利亚和新几内亚土著人中味盲者高达 42%，我国汉族人味盲者约占 9%，壮族人味盲者仅为 4%。

表 16-1　PTC 溶液浓度与个体基因型、表型的关系

PTC 溶液浓度	基因型	表型
<1/768 000	TT	纯合尝味者
1/48 000~1/384 000	Tt	杂合尝味者
>1/24 000	tt	味盲

研究表明，味盲（tt）者易患结节性甲状腺肿，因此，可将 PTC 的尝味能力检测作为该病的一种辅助诊断手段。

2. 人类的各种遗传性状是由特定基因控制形成的，每个人的遗传基础不同，某种性状在不同个体会出现不同的表现。通过特定人群的某一性状的调查，可以初步了解该性状的遗传方式、控制性状形成的基因性质，并可根据 Hardy-Weinberg 定律计算相应的基因频率、基因型频率及基因突变率。

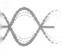

【实验步骤】

（一）PTC 尝味能力检测及分析

1. 配制梯度 PTC 溶液 称取 0.13g PTC（苯硫脲）溶于 100ml 蒸馏水中，此为 PTC 原液（饱和液），标为 0 号液，浓度为 1/750；然后取 0 号液 50ml，加蒸馏水 50ml 稀释为 1 号液；以此类推，直至稀释到 13 号液，浓度为 1/6 144 000。另设置空白对照（蒸馏水）14 号液。

2. PTC 尝味能力检测 从低浓度到高浓度，用吸管吸 1~2 滴 PTC 溶液滴在受试者舌根处，令受试者徐徐咽下品味，直至有苦味感觉为止，记下此 PTC 溶液的等级号（阈值）；为准确起见，最好重复测定一次，以两次阈值相同为准。若最高浓度的 PTC 溶液也尝不出苦味，则取少许 PTC 粉末放在舌根上，检测有无苦涩味。

3. PTC 尝味能力分析 根据受试者的尝味阈值，确定其基因型：尝味阈值低于 10 号液浓度（1/768 000）者为纯合尝味者，基因型为 TT；尝味阈值在 6 号液（1/48 000）~9 号液浓度（1/384 000）之间者为杂合尝味者，基因型为 Tt；尝味阈值高于 5 号液（1/24 000）浓度者为味盲，基因型为 tt。最后，将全班同学尝味结果记录在表中（表 16-2），计算 T、t 基因频率和 TT、Tt、tt 基因型频率。

表 16-2 PTC 尝味能力统计表（示意）

序号	姓名	性别	民族	PTC 尝味能力（PTC 溶液浓度—基因型）														
				tt						Tt				TT			
				0	1	2	3	4	5	6	7	8	9	10	11	12	13
1																	
2																	
…																	
n																	
合计																	

（二）人类部分遗传性状分析

同学之间相互观察以下遗传性状，了解其遗传方式，统计全班同学各对相对性状中不同性状的出现频率；调查家族中各性状的遗传情况，绘出系谱图，印证其遗传方式。

1. 单睑和重睑 人群中的眼睑（eyelid）可分为单睑（俗称单眼皮）和重睑（俗称双眼皮）两种性状（图 16-1）。一般认为双眼皮受显性基因控制，为显性性状；单眼皮为隐性性状。

2. 耳垂的有无 根据人类耳郭外缘下部与头部皮肤相连处是否光滑，区分为有耳垂和无耳垂（图 16-2）。耳垂部分无弹性软骨，仅含结缔组织和脂肪。有耳垂为常染色体显性遗传，无耳垂为常染色体隐性遗传。

3. 能否卷舌 卷舌是指舌的两侧能在口腔中向上卷成槽状，甚至卷成筒状，多数人有此特征，此为显性遗传；少数人不具有卷舌能力，频率约为 1‰，属隐性遗传（图 16-3）。

4. 直发和卷发 人类的发式有卷发和直发之分（图 16-4）。东方人多为直发，为隐性性状；卷发者很少，为显性性状。

5. 顺时发旋和逆时发旋 人的头顶稍后方中线处有一个发旋（有的人不止一个），其螺

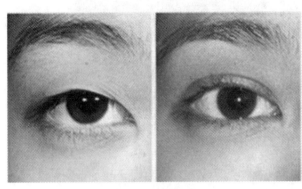

图 16-1　单睑和重睑

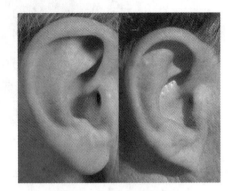

图 16-2　有耳垂与无耳垂

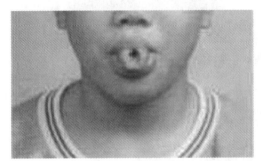

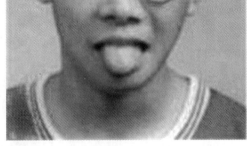

图 16-3　能否卷舌

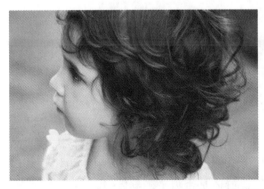

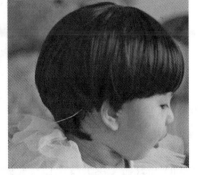

图 16-4　卷发和直发

旋方向受遗传因素控制,顺时针方向者为显性性状,逆时针方向者为隐性性状(图 16-5)。

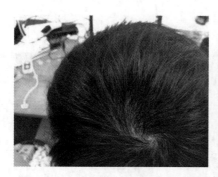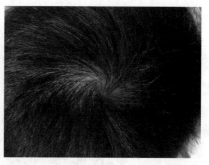

图 16-5　顺时发旋和逆时发旋

6. 峰形发际与平线发际　人群中,有些人额前发际基本呈平线状,有些人额前发际正中部分向前下延伸呈峰形,形成 V 形。峰形发际属显性遗传,平线发际属隐性遗传(图 16-6)。

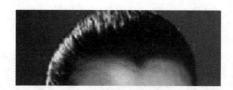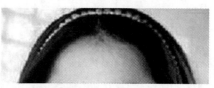

图 16-6　峰形发际与平线发际

7. 拇指关节能否超伸展　大多数人拇指末节不能向拇指背侧弯曲,少数人拇指末节能向拇指背侧弯曲,与拇指垂直轴呈 60° 角(图 16-7),称为超伸展,此性状为隐性性状。

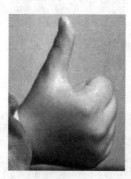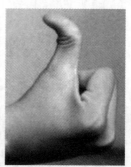

图 16-7　拇指关节能否超伸展

【分析思考】

1. β 地中海贫血是一种不完全显性遗传病,在一个 10 000 人的群体中,发现重型 β 地中海贫血患者($\beta^0\beta^0$)16 人,杂合子患者($\beta^A\beta^0$)380 人,正常人($\beta^A\beta^A$)为 9 604 人,求这一群体正常基因 β^A 和贫血基因 β^0 的频率,并判定该群体是否为平衡群体。

2. 在丹麦,矮人(显性矮化)的频率为 10.7×10^{-5},其适合度为 0.196,求矮化基因的突变率。

3. 人类全色盲为 AR 遗传,大约 8 万人中有 1 个全色盲患者,患者的子女数约为正常人的一半。求由正常基因突变为全色盲基因的频率。

4. 莱-奈恩综合征是人类神经系统的单基因遗传病(XR),调查了某地区 500 名高加索男性,发现 20 人患此病,此病的适合度为 0.15。问:①该群体正常等位基因频率和致病基因突变率各是多少? ②该地区的正常女性占多大比例?

5. 根据自己的 PTC 尝味试验结果,推断父母 PTC 尝味能力。

【实验报告】

记录全班同学 PTC 尝味能力和其他各种遗传性状的调查结果,计算相应基因的基因频率及基因型频率。

实验 17　人类遗传病分析

【目的要求】

1. 通过绘制、分析遗传病系谱及推算再发风险,熟悉遗传性疾病的基本分析方法,掌握单基因遗传病的遗传方式及其特点。

2. 熟悉多基因遗传病再发风险估计的方法。

3. 熟悉人类染色体 G 带带型特征,掌握染色体核型分析方法。

4. 了解主要染色体病的核型及异常核型的识别、描述方法。

5. 学习利用人类孟德尔遗传的网上资源——人类孟德尔遗传在线(Online Mendelian Inheritance in Man,OMIM),查阅人类遗传性状或遗传病相关资料的方法。

【实验原理】

1. 系谱分析(pedigree analysis)　是分析遗传病常用的方法。从患有某种遗传病的先证者入手,追溯调查其所有家族成员(包括直系亲属和旁系亲属)是否患该种遗传病;将调查资料以特定符号和格式绘制出反映家族各成员相互关系和发病情况的图(即系谱图);根据孟德尔遗传定律对各成员的表型和基因型进行分析,判断该遗传病的遗传方式(单基因遗传、多基因遗传);如果是单基因遗传,再进一步分析是常染色体遗传或性染色体遗传;是显性遗传、隐性遗传或 X 连锁遗传。

2. 多基因遗传病再发风险的相关因素　包括:多基因遗传病的遗传率和群体发病率,家庭中患病人数,患病成员的病情严重程度,群体发病率的性别差异等。

3. 染色体病　是染色体畸变所产生的疾病。染色体畸变包括染色体数目异常和结构畸变,前者比后者更常见;染色体断裂和断裂后的异常接合是染色体结构畸变的基础,常见的染色体结构畸变有缺失、环状染色体、易位、重复、倒位和等臂染色体等。

4. 人类孟德尔遗传学(Mendelian Inheritance in Man,MIM)　是一个数据库,该数据库对现时所知的遗传病进行分类。利用该数据库的网上资源——人类孟德尔遗传在线(Online Mendelian Inheritance in Man,OMIM)可以很方便地查找有关人类一般遗传性状或遗传病的相关资料。

【实验用品】

1. 唐氏综合征患者 G 显带染色体标本片。

2. Klinefelter 综合征患者 G 显带染色体标本片。

3. Turner 综合征患者 G 显带染色体标本片。

4. 2 号染色体与 5 号染色体相互易位患者 G 显带染色体标本片。

5. 异常染色体核型照片,核型分析表。

【实验步骤】

（一）单基因遗传病系谱分析

根据题目中给出的条件,绘出系谱图,判断遗传病的遗传方式;对所提供系谱,运用单基因遗传规律,分析讨论题目提出的问题,判断基因型,预测某些个体发病与否及发病的可能性等。

1. 一例遗传性小脑性运动失调系谱如下(图 17-1):①试判断遗传方式并说明依据。②写出患者及其父母的基因型。③为什么Ⅱ₄及其后代中没有患者? Ⅱ₄的子女如和正常人结婚,会不会生出患病的后代?

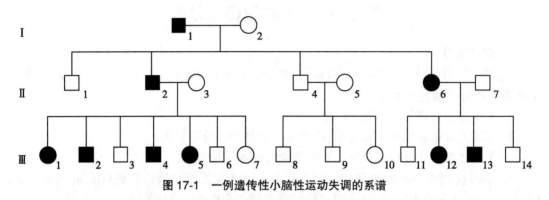

图 17-1 一例遗传性小脑性运动失调的系谱

2. 分析 α 地中海贫血的系谱(图 17-2),在括号内写出相应个体的基因型,如Ⅲ₃与群体中一轻型 α 地中海贫血患者结婚,所生出子女基因型和表现型如何?

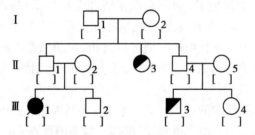

图 17-2 一例地中海贫血的系谱

注:●为 Hb Barts 胎儿水肿综合征患者,◐为 Hb H 病患者。

3. 分析图 17-3 遗传病系谱的遗传方式,在括号内写出相应个体的基因型。

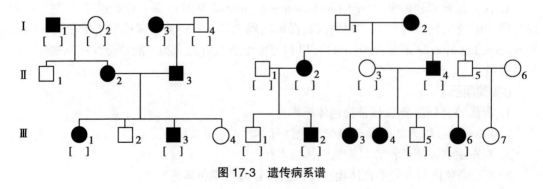

图 17-3 遗传病系谱

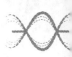

4. 已知某 AD 病外显率为 80%。在该病系谱(图 17-4)中,表型正常的女性(Ⅱ$_4$)已生育两个正常男孩,问再生出患儿的可能性多大?

5. 一对夫妇,身体健康,结婚 6 年,生有一男一女,但均因患先天性肌迟缓而死亡,为此来医院咨询。询问病史后得知,这对夫妇系表亲婚配,丈夫的父亲与妻子的母亲为兄妹俩,丈夫有一个哥哥,婚后生有一个正常女儿。据此,请绘制系谱,并判断该病的遗传方式。

6. 一对夫妇带一名 5 岁男孩就诊,男孩的症状表现为行走笨拙,摇摆,似"鸭步"状。询问病史得知,妻子的哥哥在 5 岁左右时也呈现以上症状,10 岁时肌肉萎缩,瘫痪在床,20 岁死亡。试绘出该系谱,并判断该病的遗传方式。

7. 在图 17-5 的遗传病系谱中,如Ⅱ$_3$和Ⅲ$_1$婚配,常染色体基因和 X 染色体基因的近婚系数各是多少? 如Ⅰ$_1$的等位基因组合是 Aa,Ⅱ$_3$与Ⅲ$_1$同有Ⅰ$_1$之 a 基因的概率是多少?

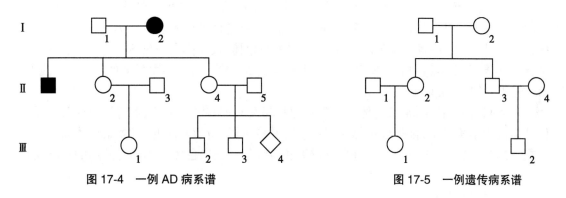

图 17-4　一例 AD 病系谱　　　　　图 17-5　一例遗传病系谱

8. 苯丙酮尿症是一种常染色体隐性遗传病,群体发病率约 1/20 000。一个人表型正常,其外甥患有此病,他如果与群体中的女性随机婚配,所生后代患苯丙酮尿症的风险如何? 他如果与他的姨表妹结婚,所生后代患苯丙酮尿症的风险又如何?

(二)多基因遗传病分析

唇裂是一种多基因遗传病,我国的群体发病率为 0.17%,遗传率为 76%,一男性患者与一正常女性结婚,所生子女患病风险多大?

(三)染色体病分析

1. 染色体病 G 显带染色体标本片观察

(1)唐氏综合征:本病是最常见的常染色体病,临床特征包括智力低下、伸舌、鼻梁低平、外眼角上斜、小耳、小颌、枕平、内眦赘皮、颈短及肌张力减低等;常伴有先天性心脏发育缺陷,急性淋巴性和粒细胞性白血病的发生率增高;发病率与母亲生育年龄呈正相关。常见核型为三体型 47,XX(XY),+21,少数为易位型或嵌合型。

观察唐氏综合征患者 G 显带染色体标本片:低倍镜下可看到大量染成蓝紫色的圆形细胞核,还可看到棒状、杆状和颗粒状结构相对集中的区域,这是一个细胞的全部染色体构成的中期分裂象。换用高倍镜,寻找分散好、互不交叉、长短合适的中期分裂象;最后用油镜观察,计数染色体数目,根据带型特征,鉴别出 21 号和性染色体(XY)。

注意:游离型患者的染色体标本片,镜下可看到 3 条 21 号染色体;而易位型患者的标本片,两条染色体易位形成的易位染色体需要仔细观察、辨认。镜下会发现 21 号染色体和 14 号染色体形成的易位染色体。

(2)Klinefelter 综合征:本病是性染色体数目异常引起的疾病,常见核型为性染色体三

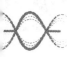

体型(47,XXY),少数为嵌合型。观察 Klinefelter 综合征患者 G 显带染色体标本片。

（3）Turner 综合征:本病是性染色体数目异常引起的疾病,常见核型为性染色体单体型(45,X),此外还有嵌合型和结构异常的核型。观察 Turner 综合征患者 G 显带染色体标本片。

（4）2 号染色体与 5 号染色体相互易位:染色体易位有多种类型,相互易位最多见,即两条染色体分别发生一次断裂,相互交换片段后重接,结果形成两条衍生染色体。观察 2 号染色体与 5 号染色体相互易位患者 G 显带染色体标本片。

2. 异常染色体核型照片剪贴分析　结构异常的染色体核型照片剪贴方法与正常 G 显带染色体核型照片剪贴方法相似,首先计数照片上染色体数目;然后根据各组染色体的结构特征,依次找出 A、B、D、E、F、G 组,剩余的为 C 组,在每条染色体旁用铅笔标出组号;不能配对的染色体,暂时放在一边,留待最后根据异常特点确定其归属;用剪刀将每条染色体连同组号剪下,放入培养皿中并计数,证实染色体全部剪下;根据 G 带的带纹特征,在每一组内进行同源染色体配对,标出染色体序号,确定不能配对染色体的序号及异常类型;最后,将染色体组号、序号剪去,将各号染色体,包括结构异常染色体,按序排在染色体核型分析表的相应位置上,用糨糊贴牢。粘贴时,使染色体的短臂居上、长臂居下,并使着丝粒处在一条直线上。剪贴过程要细心,防止丢失染色体。

未能配对的结构异常染色体常见类型包括相互易位、缺失、倒位、等臂染色体等。无论何种染色体结构异常,都是染色体断裂、断片、易位、重接所致。因此,寻找染色体断裂点很重要。判断断裂点,必须制备具有高分辨率和清晰带型的染色体标本和对照用的标准模式图,确定断裂点发生的具体带或亚带。

3. 异常核型的描述

（1）染色体数目异常的核型描述:根据人类细胞遗传学命名的国际体制(ISCN),染色体数目异常的核型描述,用染色体总数、性染色体组成、增加或减少的染色体序号及染色体序号前的"+"或"–"表示,如 47,XX,+21。

（2）染色体结构畸变核型的描述:分为简式和详式两种。简式用染色体总数、性染色体组成、结构畸变的符号、结构畸变染色体的序号及染色体上断裂点的位置表示,后两项均写在括号内,例如 46,XX,t(2;5)(q21;q31)。

详式与简式的区别在于,结构畸变的染色体不是用断裂点位置表示,而是用具体描述结构畸变染色体带的构成,上例用详式表示为 46,XX,t(2;5)(2pter → 2q21 ∶∶ 5q31 → 5qter; 5pter → 5q31 ∶∶ 2q21 → 2qter)。

（四）人类遗传资源数据库的利用

1. 熟悉 MIM 数据库的构成　MIM 数据库的资料是在 McKusick VA 博士带领下,在约翰·霍普金斯大学的一组科学工作者及编辑协助下收集和处理的。相关的文章经过鉴定、讨论,最终编写在数据库内成为相关的条目。

MIM 自 1966 年初版以来,随着医学遗传学的迅猛发展,MIM 内容急剧扩增,至 1998 年已出版至第 12 版。印刷版本的 MIM,尽管不断增厚,但在科学研究已进入数字化时代的现在,显然已很难跟上医学遗传学发展的步伐,因此,1987 年,该数据库的网上版本——人类孟德尔遗传在线(Online Mendelian Inheritance in Man,OMIM)应运而生,并且免费供全世界科学家浏览和下载,网址是 http://www.ncbi.nlm.nih.gov/omim。

MIM 包括所有已知的遗传病、遗传决定的性状及其基因,除了简略描述各种疾病的临床特征、诊断、鉴别诊断、治疗与预防外,还提供已知有关致病基因的连锁关系、染色体定位、组成结构和功能、动物模型等资料,并附有经缜密筛选的相关参考文献。在 MIM 的数据库中,人类的每种已知性状或疾病及相关基因都有一个独特的 6 位编号,简称 MIM 号,为全世界所公认,有关遗传病的报道必须冠以 MIM 号,以明确所讨论的是哪一种遗传病。

MIM 号首位是遗传方式的分类,1 代表染色体显性遗传,2 代表染色体隐性遗传,3 代表 X 连锁遗传等。在第 12 版的 MIM 中,所有编号都加上方括号;编号前的"*"代表已知的遗传方式,编号前"#"代表该病征由 2 个或 2 个以上基因突变而成。例如,佩利措伊斯 - 梅茨巴赫(Pelizaeus-Merzbacher)病(MIM*169500)就是指已知的、常染色体显性遗传病。MIM 编号范围与遗传方式的对应关系见表 17-1。

表 17-1　MIM 编号范围与遗传方式的关系

首号码	MIM 编号范围	遗传方式
1	100 000~199 999	常染色体显性位点或有关表型(1994 年 5 月 15 日前创建)
2	200 000~299 999	常染色体隐性位点或有关表型(1994 年 5 月 15 日前创建)
3	300 000~399 999	X 连锁位点或有关表型
4	400 000~499 999	Y 连锁位点或有关表型
5	500 000~599 999	线粒体位点或有关表型
6	600 000~	染色体位点或有关表型(1994 年 5 月 15 日后创建)

截至 2020 年 12 月 23 日的统计数据,OMIM 总条目数为 25 687 个,其中,常染色体遗传条目 24 243 个,X 连锁遗传条目 1 311 个,Y 连锁遗传条目 63 个,线粒体遗传条目 70 个(其中基因 37 个,有分子基础的性状 33 个)。已经定位的人类基因数目(不包括 EST、假基因、基因标志、cDNA)为 16 395 个。熟练应用 OMIM,可以很方便地查找有关人类一般遗传性状或遗传病的相关资料。

2. OMIM 的应用　进入网址 http://www.ncbi.nlm.nih.gov/omim,分别查找一种单基因病、线粒体病、多基因病、染色体病及遗传性肿瘤的有关资料,填写下列有关内容:

中文病名:

英文病名:

OMIM 编号:

基因座或涉及的染色体:

遗传方式:

群体发病率:

临床症状:

发病机制:

致病突变方式:

诊断方法(临床诊断、生化诊断或基因诊断等):

预防措施:

治疗方法:

【分析思考】

1. 人类染色体畸变包括哪些类型? 举例说明染色体畸变的核型描述方法。

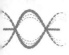

2. 某一外表正常的妇女,经染色体检查发现所有中期分裂象中都有 1 条臂间倒位的 2 号染色体,断裂点在 2p21 和 2q31,其他染色体正常。根据 ISCN(1995)的人类染色体简式和详式的描述方法,写出该妇女的核型;如该妇女与正常男性婚配,所生后代染色体核型有哪些可能性?

3. 写出下列核型形成的机制

(1) 46,XX/47,XX,+13

(2) 45,XX,t(21q21q)

(3) 46,XY,t(8;16)(p22;q21)

(4) 45,XX,-18

【实验报告】

剪贴分析一张人类异常体细胞 G 显带中期分裂象染色体照片并写出核型。

第二部分　留学生实验

（Part Ⅱ　International Student Experiments）

Experiment 18　Ordinary Optical Microscope

【Purpose and requirements】

1. Be familiar with the main structure and performance of the ordinary optical microscope.
2. To Master the use of low power objective and high power objective.
3. To learn the use of oil immersion objective initially.
4. Be familiar with maintenance methods of ordinary optical microscope.

【Experimental principle】

Optical microscope, makes small objects form magnified images using the magnifying imaging principle of convex lens illuminated by the light source. The microscope has been invented and used for more than 400 years. Around 1590, Janssen and his son in Holland developed a primitive microscope that magnified ten times. In 1665, the English physicist R. Hooke developed a better microscope and used it to discover cells. Over the past 400 years, through continuous improvement, the microscope's structure and performance have been gradually improved. At present, the commonly used is the double tube tilted microscope. Most microscopes have electrical source except for a few which use reflectors for daylighting. In addition to the ordinary optical microscopes, there are phase contrast microscopes, darkfield microscopes, fluorescence microscopes and laser scanning confocal microscopes with special functions or applications. All kinds of the optical microscopes differ significantly in shape and structure, but their basic structure and working principle are similar. An ordinary optical microscope is mainly composed of the mechanical system and optical system. The optical system as the core part of the microscope includes eyepiece, objective, condenser and reflector (or electric light source), and other components (Fig. 18-1).

Although the structure of eyepiece and objective is more complex, their function is equivalent to a convex lens. Because the test specimen is placed between 1~2 times the focal length under the objective, the objective can make specimens form a handstand magnified real image; the real image is just in the lower focus (focal plane) of the eyepiece, the eyepiece can further enlarge it into a virtual image. Through focus, the virtual image can fall on in the visual distance of eyes, thus forming a real image of upright in the retina. The magnified, inverted virtual image in the optical microscope is consistent with the upright real image on the retina, which appears to be 25cm away from the eye (Fig. 18-2).

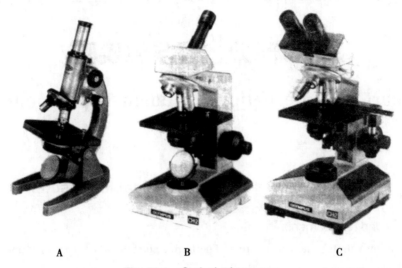

Fig. 18-1　Optical microscope

A. single cylinder upright type；B. single cylinder inclined type；C. double cylinder inclined type.

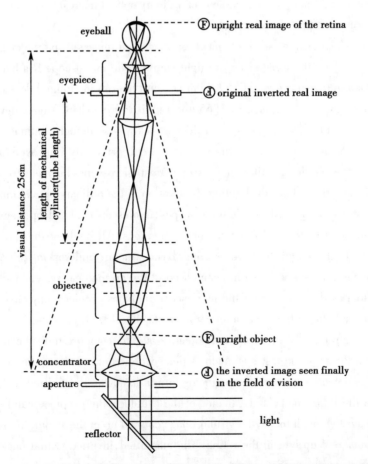

Fig. 18-2　Principle of magnification and light path diagram of the optical microscope

Resolution，magnification，aperture ratio，focal depth and field width reflect the performance and quality of optical microscope. These performance indicators have certain limits；they interact

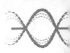

with each other, restrict each other, improve or improve one aspect of performance, and often make another performance lower.

The resolution (R) is the most critical performance index of an optical microscope. It refers to the minimum distance that can distinguish two particles on the object at the visual distance of 25cm. Therefore the smaller the resolution, the higher the resolving power. The resolution of human eyes is about 100μm, while the resolution of the optical microscope is up to 0.2μm. The resolution of the optical microscope is determined by the resolution of the objective, which is the resolution of the microscope, while the eyepiece has nothing to do with the resolution of the microscope. It only magnifies the image resolved by the objective for the second time. The resolution of optical microscope can be calculated as follows:

$$R = 0.61\lambda/N.A. = 0.61\lambda/n \cdot \sin(\alpha/2) \qquad (18\text{-}1)$$

Where λ is the lighting source's wavelength, the shortest wavelength of visible light is 0.4μm. N.A. stands for numerical aperture, also known as aperture ratio. Its value is equal to the product of the refractive index (n) of the medium between the objective and the sample to be tested and the sine value of half of the lens angle (α), that is, $N.A. = n \times \sin(\alpha/2)$. The maximum value of n is 1.5 (the medium is cedar oil). The angle of lens mouth refers to the angle formed by the light from a point on the optical axis of the objective extending to the two ends of the effective diameter of the lens in front of the objective. The larger the lens angle is, the more light enters the objective, and the maximum value of $\sin(\alpha/2)$ is 1 (α=180°). Therefore, N.A. the maximum is $n \times \sin(\alpha/2) = 1.5 \times 1 = 1.5$.

It can be seen from the above formula that the N.A. of the objective determines the main optical properties of a microscope, the larger N.A., the smaller the resolution, the stronger the resolving power of the microscope, and the better the optical performance. However, N.A. is inversely proportional to the depth of focus (that is, the distance or range of the image above and below the plane of focus when the microscope is focusing on a point or plane of the specimen), so it's not that the bigger the N.A. the better. The N.A. of the objective is usually marked on the edge of the objective.

When using low power objective and high power objective, the air is the medium, the "n" value is 1.0; when using oil immersion objective, cedar oil is the medium, the "n" value is 1.5 (maximum value of n). Therefore, the N.A. of oil immersion objective is greater than that of low power objective and high power objective; that is, the resolving power of oil immersion objective is higher than that of low power objective and high power objective. At present, the maximum N.A. of the objective (oil immersion objective) is 1.4 in the practical range. By substituting λ and N.A. into the formula for resolution calculation, we can get $R = 0.61 \times 0.4\mu m/1.4 \approx 0.174\mu m$, that is, the minimum resolution of the microscope is about 0.2μm. Besides, Due to the different densities of air and slide, when light passes through the air medium between slide and objective, scattering occurs, which reduces the illumination of the field of vision; while the refractive index of slide and cedar oil is similar, when light passes through, it almost does not refract, which increases the amount of light in the field of vision. Therefore, when the oil immersion objective is used to observe the specimen, the object image will be more clear.

Magnification is another critical parameter of the optical microscope performance. The total magnification of the optical microscope is equal to the product of eyepiece magnification and objective magnification.

This lesson mainly studies the basic structure, function and use of ordinary optical microscope (after this referred to a microscope).

【Experimental supplies】

1. Materials and Reagents   human blood smear or toad blood smear, wool cross slide, English letter slide, cedar oil (or liquid paraffin), anhydrous ethanol (or ether ethanol mixture).

2. Equipments   microscope, lens paper.

【Experimental procedures】

1. Be familiar with the basic structure and function of ordinary optical microscope

1.1   Mechanical system

1.1.1   Mirror tube: Mirror tube is a cylindrical structure mounted at the top of a microscope with an eyepiece at the top and an objective converter at the bottom (Fig. 18-3).

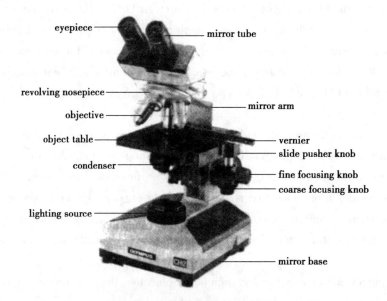

Fig. 18-3   Microscopic structure

1.1.2   Revolving nosepiece: Revolving nosepiece also known as the rotating disc or objective converter, is a disc-shaped structure installed under the mirror tube, which can rotate clockwise and counterclockwise. There are 3~4 circular holes evenly distributed on it, and the objective of different magnification can be installed. The objective converter can be rotated to make the different objectives reach the working position (that is, the axis with the light path).

1.1.3   Mirror arm: Mirror arm is a structure supporting the mirror tube and the stage. The lower end is connected with the mirror base, and it also is the part to hold when taking the microscope.

1.1.4   Focal adjuster: Focal adjuster is a device for adjusting the focal length, which is located below the mirror arm. There is a coarse focusing knob (large knob) and a fine focusing knob (small knob). The coarse focusing knob can make the object table rise and fall faster, i.e, quickly adjust the focal length, seeing the object image in the visual field; it is suitable for focusing when observing at low power objective. The fine focusing knob makes the object table rise or fall slowly, and the amplitude of the rise or fall is not easy to be observed by the naked eye; it is suitable for fine adjustment of the focal length of high power objective and oil immersion objective and observing different focal planes of the same specimen.

1.1.5   Stage: Stage is a square platform under nosepiece, which is used to place the slide specimen observed. There is a circular light hole in the center of the stage, through which the light from below shines on the specimen. A specimen moving device, also known as slide pusher, is installed on the stage. The spring clip installed on the slide pusher is used to fix the slide specimen. By rotating the two knobs of the slide pusher, the slide specimen can be moved back and forth or left and right.

A vertical and horizontal vernier is attached to the slide pusher to mark the position of the specimen. The vernier consists of the paramount ruler (A) and the sub-ruler (B), and the sub-ruler's grading is 9/10 of the paramount ruler. When using, first look at the position of 0 point of the secondary scale, and then look at the coincidence point of the main scale and the subsidiary scale; according to the coincidence point, you can read out the accurate value. The value shown in Fig. 18-4 should be 26.4.

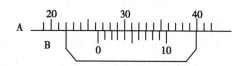

Fig. 18-4   Usage of the vernier

1.1.6   Mirror base: Mirror base is located at the bottom of the entire microscope, which is used to support and stabilize the microscope.

1.2   Optical system: The optical system includes eyepiece, objective, condenser, reflector (or electric light source), etc.

1.2.1   Eyepiece: Eyepiece is installed at the upper end of the mirror tube, which can further enlarge the object image magnified by the objective. Each microscope is usually equipped with three to four eyepieces with different magnification, such as " × 5" " × 10" and " × 15" (the number represents the magnification), which can be selected according to different needs, and the most commonly used eyepiece is the " × 10" eyepiece. To facilitate the indication of structure in the field of view, a small piece of thin wire can be attached to the field of view aperture in the eyepiece as a pointer. In addition, an eyepiece micrometer may be mounted on the field-of-view aperture.

1.2.2   Objective: Objective is mounted on an revolving nosepiece. Each microscope generally has 3 to 4 objective with different magnification, and the objective is the most critical optical component of the micros. It determines the size of the microscope's resolution. The magnification of the commonly used objective lens is " × 4" " × 10" " × 40" (or " × 45") and " × 100". Generally, the " × 4" " × 10" objective is called low power objective, the " × 40" or " × 45" objective is called a high power objective, the " × 100" objective is called oil immersion objective (the top of this objective needs to be immersed in cedar oil or liquid paraffin wax when it is used). The peripheral of each objective is usually marked with parameters that can reflect its main performance (Fig. 18-5), including magnification and numerical aperture (e.g, 10/0.25, 40/0.65, and 100/1.25), the length of the mirror tube and the coverslip thickness (160/0.17, mm) required for the objective. Besides, the oil immersion objective is often marked with "oil".

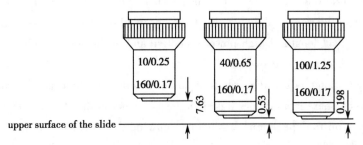

Fig. 18-5 Performance parameters and a working distance of the objective

Note: The distance between the two arrows is the working distance, unit: mm.

Different objective have different working distances. The so-called working distance refers to the distance between the bottom end of the objective and the upper surface of the coverslip when the microscope is in operation (the focal length is well adjusted and the image is clear) (Fig. 18-5). The magnification of the objective is inversely proportional to its working distance.

When the low power objective is adjusted to the working distance, it can be directly converted into high power objective or oil immersion objective, then you only need to rotate the fine focusing knob to see a clear image. Different magnification of the objective can be distinguished from the shape. Generally, the low power objective is the shortest, the oil immersion objective is the longest, and the high power objective length between the two.

1.2.3　Condenser: Condenser is located under the light hole on the stage. Its primary function is to focus the light on the specimen to be observed. The condenser consists of two or three lenses, which act as a convex lens and concentrate the light into a beam. There is usually an adjusting knob at the lower left of the condenser, also known as the adjusting handle of the aperture diaphragm of the condenser, which is used to lift or lower the condenser. Raising the condenser will increase the light, otherwise, the light will become weaker.

1.2.4　Aperture: Aperture is located under the condenser, and is composed of a group of metal sheets. A small handle on the outside of the aperture is moved to make the aperture larger or smaller to adjust light intensity. Some microscopes have a filter frame below the aperture to place filters of different colors.

1.2.5　Reflector: Reflector is located below the condenser and can be rotated in all directions to reflect light from different directions into the condenser. The reflector has a plane and a concave: concave has the function of light concentration, suitable for weak light and scattered light use; when the light is intense, the plane is chosen. For the electric light source microscope, the dimming knob is used to adjust the brightness.

2. Learn how to use the microscope

2.1　low power objective

2.1.1　preparing: When moving the double cylinder inclined type microscope, hold the mirror arm with the right hand and hold the mirror seat with the left hand. Place the microscope smoothly on the experimental bench in front of your seat. The rear edge of the mirror base is 3~6cm away from the experimental bench's edge. Handle with care. Adjust the height of the stool so that your eyes can view the eyepiece comfortably.

2.1.2　Dimming：First，rotate the coarse-focusing knob to lower the stage slightly；then，rotate nosepiece to make the low power objective rotate in place（that is，the low power objective is aimed at the light hole）；when the objective is fully in place，a slight tumbling sound can be heard. Open the aperture wide，raise the condenser to the appropriate position（the lens plane above the condenser is slightly lower than the plane of the stage is appropriate），and turn the concave surface of the reflector to the light source；then，look at the eyepiece with both eyes，and adjust the angle of the reflector so that the light in the field of vision is uniform and moderately bright. If an electric optical microscope is used，the dimming screw is used to adjust the brightness.

2.1.3　Place the slide：Take the slide specimen that needs to be observed，first observe it with naked eyes in front of the light to understand the whole picture of the specimen；then，put the slide with the coverslip side up on the stage，and fix it with the spring clamp on the slide pusher；finally，rotate the slide pusher knob to make the part that needs to be observed in the center of the light hole.

2.1.4　Focusing：While looking at the distance between the low power objective and the slide from the side with eyes，at the same time，adjust the coarse-focus knob to rise the stage until the distance between the low power objective and the slide specimen is about 0.5cm；then，both eyes observe from the eyepiece and slowly turn the coarse focusing knob to lower the stage until the object image appears in the field of vision. Finally，turn the fine focusing knob to make the object image in the field of view clear. This state is called the quasi-focus state，and the process of focusing is called the quasi-focus. Each person's binocular pupil distance is different. By adjusting the distance between the two eyepiece axis，the field of view coincides to form a complete circular field of view. When focusing，if the distance between the objective and the slide has been more than 1cm and the object image is still not seen，the reason should be found and corrected：① If the objective is not fully rotated in place，or the lens is not aligned with the light hole，the objective should be rotated in place before observation；② If the specimen is out of the field of vision，the slide pusher should be moved so that the specimen moves to the center of the field of vision；③ If the coarse-focusing knob rotates too fast and exceeds the focus，the coarse-focusing knob should be rotated slowly；④ If the light in the field of vision is too strong or the specimen is lightly stained or the specimen is not stained，the light should be appropriately dimmed. Whatever the reason，re-focus precisely as described above.

2.2　high power objective

2.2.1　Select observation target：Before using the high power objective，you should first use the low power objective to find the object for further observation and move it to the center of the vision field.

2.2.2　Change to high power objective：To prevent the objective from colliding with the slide，when rotating the nosepiece，watch from the side of the microscope and slowly rotate the high power objective into place；that is，the high power objective is aimed at the light hole.

2.2.3　Focusing：After the high power objective is rotated in place，the object image that

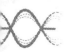

is not very clear can be seen in the field of vision. At this point, the object image is clear by just slightly adjusting the fine focusing knob. If the field of vision is not bright enough, you can raise the condenser, open the aperture and adjust the angle of the reflector (electric light source microscope can increase the brightness).

If the objective touches the slide when changing the high power objective, it should not be forced to rotate at this time. The reason should be found and corrected. Common reasons include: ① The bottom of the slide is up; ② the slide is too thick; ③ high power objective loosening; ④ low power objective is not focused, etc. If the high power objective still touches the slide after eliminating these factors, it means that the high power objective is too long, and it may be a non original high power objective. At this case, the stage should be lowered and converted to the high power objective first; then, under the gaze of the eyes, slowly raise the stage until the high power objective approaches the coverslip; finally, while observing the eyepiece, the stage is lowered slowly with coarse-focusing knob, after seeing the object image, then use fine focusing knob quasi-focus.

Due to manufacturing technology, there is always a certain deviation between the center of the field of vision of low power and that of high power objective with many microscopes. Therefore, it is often difficult for the observer to quickly find the specimen when switching from low power objective to high power objective. This problem can be solved by drawing an eccentricity diagram. The specific approach is: first find the wool crossing point at the high power objective and move it to the center of the field of vision, then change the low power objective to observe the wool crossing point in the field vision, where is the eccentric position. Repeat the operation several times, find out the accurate eccentric position and draw the eccentric map. Before viewing the specimen with the high power objective, the object to be further magnified should be moved to eccentric position on the low power objective, and then converted to the high power objective viewing so that the object to be observed is exactly in the center of the field of view.

2.3　Oil immersion objective

2.3.1　Select observation target: Move the object observed at low power objective or high power objective and requiring further magnification to the center of the field of vision.

2.3.2　Dimming　Raise the condenser to a higher position and open the aperture to the maximum (the oil immersion objective requires intense light).

2.3.3　Change to Oil immersion objective: Turn the revolving nosepiece and remove the low power objective or high power objective; drop a drop of cedar oil (or liquid paraffin) on the part of the light hole in the slide specimen, and under the gaze of the eyes, turn the oil immersion objective in place; at this time the lower end of the oil immersion objective should just be immersed in or contact with the oil drops. In some microscopes, the oil immersion objective is too long to be turn in place. At this time, you can first slightly drop the stage and then turn the oil immersion objective into place so that the lower end of the oil immersion objective is immersed in the oil droplets.

2.3.4　Focusing: While viewing the eyepiece with both eyes, carefully and slowly turn the fine focusing knob to lower the stage until a clear object image appears in the field of view. Do not turn the fine focusing knob in the opposite direction during operation, lest the lens crushes the specimen or damages the lens.

In the process of using the oil immersion objective to observe, if it is necessary to replace the observation target, in order to prevent the high power objective from getting with oil, the oil immersion objective can be directly replaced after the low power objective observes a certain target.

2.3.5　Cleaning: After the end of oil immersion objective use, the oil (or liquid paraffin) on the lens must be wiped clean in time. Before wiping an oil immersion objective, it should be turned away from the light hole, wipe 2 times first with a lens paper moistened with a little anhydrous ethanol (or ethyl ether ethanol mixture) and 1 time then with a lens paper. The oil (or liquid paraffin) on the slide also needs to be treated cleanly, In the case of a permanent slide specimen with coverslip, it may be wiped directly with the above described method of wiping oil immersion objective; if it is a specimen without coverslip, remove the oil (or liquid paraffin) on the slide by paper pulling method, that is, first cover a small piece of lens paper on the surface of the coverslip, then drop a few drops of anhydrous ethanol (or ethyl ether ethanol mixture) on the lens paper, and pull the lens paper to one side as soon as possible, so the oil (or liquid paraffin) on the slide can be removed by repeating this for several times.

2.4　Attention tips

2.4.1　When taking the microscope, it should be handled with care. Hold the mirror arm with one hand and hold the mirror base with the other. Do not use a single hand to avoid parts slipping.

2.4.2　The microscope should not be placed on the edge of the experimental bench. The rear edge of the lens seat should be 3~6cm away from the experimental bench's edge. When leaving your seat during the class break, the microscope should be returned to the non working state, and the objective should be turned away from the light hole.

2.4.3　Do not disassemble the parts on the microscope at will to avoid loss or damage; do not take out the eyepiece at will to prevent dust from falling into the mirror tube.

2.4.4　Always keep the microscope clean. The optical parts of the microscope can only be gently wiped with the lens paper and can not be wiped with gauze, handkerchief, ordinary paper, or fingers, so as to avoid wearing the lens.

2.4.5　Using the high power objective and oil immersion objective for observation, only fine focusing knob can be adjusted. If the coarse focusing knob is turned to raise the stage, it is easy to cause the objective to collide with the slide and damage the objective or slide sample. When the specimen needs to be replaced, the coarse focusing knob should be turned first to descend the stage, so that the distance between objective and the stage is extended, and then remove the slide.

2.4.6　If you need to discuss a particular structure in the field of vision with the teacher or students, you can use the slide pusher to move the structure to the tip of the pointer; if there is no pointer in the mirror, the field of view can be seen as a clock face with a scale around (such as 3:00, 6:00, 9:00, 12:00, etc.), indicating that the structure is located in the clock face at what time position.

2.4.7　After the use of the microscope, it should be restored in time: first, lower the stage, remove the slide specimen, and turn the objective away from the light hole; then, the stage is raised, so that the objective lens is close to the stage. Put the reflector in the vertical position (or turn off the power), lower the condenser, and turn off the aperture. Finally, return the microscope to the

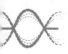

microscope room.

　　3. Operation exercises

　　3.1　Observing English letters slide, wool cross slide, or other specimens slides: When viewing English letters slide, first observe the orientation and size of letters directly with the naked eye, and then observe them under low power objective. What happens to the orientation of the letters in the field of view? How does the direction of movement of the specimen differ from the direction of movement of the object in the field of vision?

　　When observing the wool cross slide, first carefully observe the intersection point of two wool under the low power objective, then move the intersection point to the center of the field of vision, and observe by high power objective. The fine focusing knob is used to focus the two wool separately, and the up and down positions of the two wool are distinguished. If there is a deviation between low power objective and high power objective visual field center, it can be solved by drawing an eccentricity diagram as described above.

　　3.2　Observing human blood smear or toad blood smear: The blood film on the human blood smear is bluish-purple after being stained with Wright's staining; the bluish-purple blood film is aim at the light hole, on low power objective, a large number of dense red blood cells, a small number of scattered white blood cells and platelets can be seen. After careful observation with high power objective or oil immersion objective, it can be seen that erythrocytes are anucleate and centrally pale; white blood cells all have nuclei with different shapes; platelets are small and irregularly shaped (Fig. 18-6).

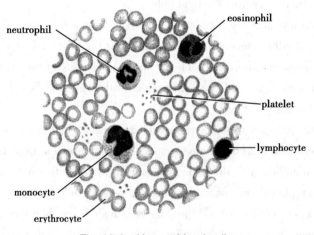

Fig. 18-6　Human blood cells

　　3.3　Observing toad spinal cord transverse slice Microscopically: The motor nerve cells in the spinal cord's anterior horn are irregular, mostly triangular or star-shaped; the cytoplasm was stained blue-purple, with a round nucleus in the center, and large and round nucleoli in some nuclei; the protrusions of the cell soma extending toward the periphery are dendrites. The small cells with darker staining are glial cells.

【 Analysis and thinking 】

1. Why is it necessary to observe specimens with a microscope in the order from low power

objective to high power objective and then to oil immersion objective?

2. Why should the distance between the low power objective and the specimen surface be adjusted to 0.5cm before focusing? While for oil immersion objective to focus, first make the oil immersion objective close to the surface of the specimen?

3. If the specimen slide is placed upside down, can the object image be found with high power objective or oil immersion objective?

4. What should you do if the structure seen at low power objective can't be found at high power objective?

5. How can you accurately and quickly find a target at high power objective?

6. What should you do if the fine focusing knob has been turned to the limit while the object image is still unclear?

7. How is the source of the stains seen in the field of vision judged? What role does an eyepiece play in microscopic imaging?

【Experimental report】

Label the names of the microscope parts in Fig. 18-7.

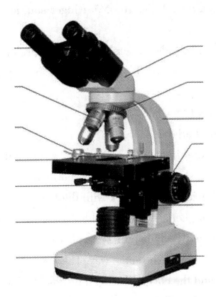

Fig. 18-7　Microscope components

Experiment 19　Basic Morphology and Structure of Cell

【Purpose and requirements】

1. To learn the method of killing toad.

2. To master the production technology of temporary slides.

3. Be familiar with the basic morphology and structure of animal and plant cells under the optical microscope.

4. To learn the method of biological drawing.

5. Be familiar with the use of commonly used anatomical equipment.

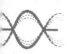

【Experimental principle】

1. Temporary specimen slide is a kind of specimen prepared on the spot from the material used for microscope observation. The temporary specimen's material is a living tissue or cell obtained from an organism, which can be observed by microscope after staining. According to the material's source and structure, the temporary specimen slide includes laying, smear, tabletting, etc. It is a common method to observe cell morphology and basic structure.

2. The morphology and structure of cells are closely related to their function, especially in highly differentiated cells. For example, the muscle cells with contractile function are slender, the nerve cells with the function of sensing stimuli and conducting impulses have dendritic processes of different lengths, the red blood cells of mammals are doubly concave disc-shaped. Although different cells have different shapes, most cells include three parts: plasma membrane, cytoplasm, and nucleus under optical microscope, with a few specialized exceptions, such as the disappearance of the nucleus after maturation of mammalian erythrocytes.

【Experimental supplies】

1. Materials and reagents   Onion, toad, human oral mucosal epithelial cells, 0.2% methylene blue, 1% toluidine blue, 1% iodine solution, 0.65% Ringer solution (amphibians), Wright's dye, normal saline.

2. Equipments   Microscope, slide, coverslip, lens paper, cleaning gauze, absorbent paper, sterilized toothpick, knife, dissecting needle, tweezers, scissors, ophthalmic scissors, petri dish, pipette.

【Experimental procedures】

1. Human oral mucosal epithelial cells

1.1   Making temporary specimen slide: Drop 0.2% methylene blue dye (or 1% iodine solution) on one end of the clean slide and one drop of normal saline on the other end, then gently scrape the oral mucosa on the inside of the cheek with the blunt end of the sterilized toothpick, put the toothpick containing epithelial cells parallel in the dye on the slide, roll back and forth several times, so that the cells fall into the dye and stain 2~3min. Take another toothpick and make the oral epithelial cells fall into normal saline in the same way. The coverslip are covered at both ends of the slide. If there is excess dye around the coverslip, it can be absorbed with absorbent paper.

1.2   Microscopic examination: When observing the stained specimen in one end, the low power objective was used to look for the cells. It can be seen that the oral mucosal epithelial cells are stained blue (yellowish-brown with iodine staining) in groups or scattered. The well-dispersed cells are selected and observed with high power objective, the cells are oblate oval, polygonal, or irregular. The oval nucleus is located in the center, stained dark blue (or dark yellowish-brown), and dark nucleoli can be seen in some nuclei. The cytoplasm is uniform, dyed light blue (or light yellow), and particles of different sizes in the cytoplasm can be seen after fine focusing (Fig. 19-1).

Observe the unstained specimen at the other end of the slide, and what is the difference between the stained specimen and the unstained specimen? When observing unstained specimens, how can the brightness of the visual field be adjusted to obtain good observation?

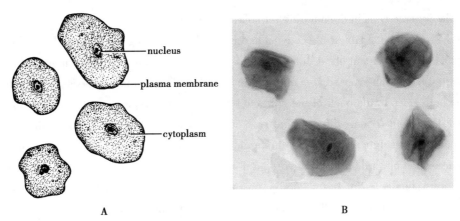

Fig.19-1　Epithelial cells from human oral mucosa

A. Pattern diagram; B. Microstructure diagram.

2. Onion epidermis cell

2.1　Making temporary specimen slide: Take a clean slide and drop a drop 1% iodine solution; cut the onion bulb into small pieces with a knife, take a fleshy scale leaf, cut it into small pieces of 3~4mm^2 with scissors; then gently tear off its inner surface with tweezers and place it in the dye of the slide. After dyeing for 2~3min, cover the coverslip and absorb the excess dye around the coverslip with absorbent paper.

2.2　Microscopic examination: At low power objective, many long rhomboidal cells arranged neatly and connected with each other can be seen. There is a thick cell wall on the cell surface, which is the main feature of plant cells. The plasma membrane can not be distinguished because it is close to the cell wall. At high power objective, the nucleus is oval, mostly located in the center of the cell and stained yellow, whereas the nucleus of mature cells is often located at the edge of the cell due to the squeeze of vacuoles. Turning the fine focusing knob, it can be seen that there are 1~2 dark yellow nucleoli with strong refraction in the nucleus. One or several vacuoles and fine particles can be seen in the cytoplasm (Fig 19-2).

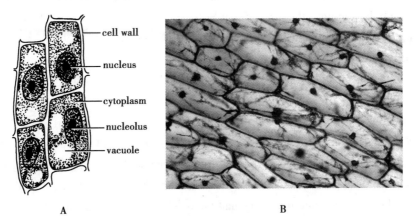

Fig. 19-2　Epidermal cells of onion bulbs

A. Pattern diagram; B. Microstructure diagram.

3. Motor nerve cells in the anterior horn of the toad spinal cord

3.1　Preparation of tabletting：One toad sacrificed by disrupting the brain and spinal cord（see appendix）, the head was cut off at the oral fissure, the medulla oblongata was removed; the scissors were inserted into at the exposed area of the spinal canal, and the spinal canal was cut longitudinally along the both sides of the back of the spine to expose the milky spinal cord. First, cut the middle spinal cord of about 0.5cm with surgical scissors, put it in a petri dish, wash off the blood with amphibious Ringer solution and absorb the liquid with absorbent paper; then put the washed spinal cord cross-section upward on the slide, drop a drop of 1% toluidine blue dye on the specimen, stain about 3~5min; finally, cover the coverslip, press down the specimen with the ventral side of the thumb, absorb the spilled dye with absorbent paper, and continue to dye 5~10min.

3.2　Microscopic examination：Microscopically, the motor nerve cells in the spinal cord's anterior horn are irregular, mostly triangular or star-shaped; the cytoplasm was stained blue-purple, with round nucleus in the center, and large and round nucleoli in some nuclei; multiple elongated protrusions of the cell soma extending toward the periphery are dendrites. The small cells with darker staining around the motor nerve cells in the spinal cord's anterior horn are glial cells（Fig 19-3）.

Fig. 19-3　Motor neurons of the anterior horn of the spinal cord

4. Toad hepatocyte

4.1　Preparation of tabletting：Cut the toad's chest-abdomen cavity to expose the dark red liver, cut off a piece of tissue about 2mm^3 at the edge of the liver, and put it in a petri dish（note that the tissue block must not be too large）. Wash with amphibian Ringer solution, gently squeeze the blood out of the liver tissue with tweezers, then put it on the slide, further cut the liver tissue into pieces with ophthalmic scissors, discard the larger pieces of tissue, drop a drop of 0.2% methylene blue dye for 3~5min, cover the coverslip, gently tap the coverslip with the handle of the dissecting needle, and continue staining 5~10min.

4.2　Microscopic examination：Microscopically, the hepatocytes were closely arranged; looking for individual hepatocyte or nonoverlapping hepatocytes, it can be seen that the hepatocytes appear polygonal, with the nuclei stained blue; note the shape and number of nuclei.

5. Toad blood cell

5.1　preparation of blood smear：Cut a small incision in the toad's heart, suck the blood with a pipette, drop one drop on the right end of the slide, place one end of the other slide on the left side of the drop, then move right to contact with the drop, and make the drop spread out along its edge; finally, the other slide is pushed smoothly to the left end of the slide at an angle of 30°~45°. When pushing the slide, press the slide tightly against the one below, move a little faster, and dry at room temperature（Fig. 19-4）.

5.2　Dyeing：Take the dried blood smear, draw a circle with a crayon in the area where the blood film is thin and uniform, and add a few drops of Wright's dye inside the circle. After about 1 min, dilute the dye with the same amount of distilled water and continue to dye 2~3 min. Rinse the dye with tap water and dry it for microscopic examination.

5.3　Microscopic examination: At low power objective, many red blood cells, and a few white blood cells can be seen. At high power objective, red blood cells are oval and nucleated, while white nuclei are round and purplish-blue (Fig. 19-5).

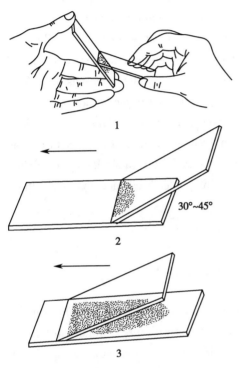

Fig. 19-4　Method for preparation of blood smears

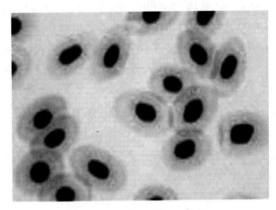

Fig. 19-5　Toad blood cells

【 Analysis and thinking 】

1. To illustrate the morphological and structural characteristics of motor nerve cells and hepatocytes in the toad spinal cord's anterior horn, and to compare the similarities and differences between them.

2. To illustrate the similarities and differences in morphology and structure between human red blood cells and toad red blood cells.

【 Experimental report 】

1. Draw structural map of human oral mucosal epithelial cells under high power objective.

2. Draw morphology and structure of onion cells under high power objective.

3. Draw morphology and structure of motor nerve cells in the anterior horn of toad spinal cord under high power objective.

【 Supplement 】Cell biology drawing methods and basic requirements

Cell biology mapping is an accurate description of the cell structure observed under the optical microscope. The drawing methods and requirements are as follows:

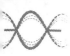

1. Reasonable layout and moderate size. Considering that the name and magnification of the drawing should be marked at the bottom of the diagram, and the structure name should be marked on the right side of the diagram, the drawing area (that is, the position of the diagram) should be slightly above and slightly to the left.

2. The drawing must be true and accurate. Careful observation of the structures under the microscope should be taken before drawing. The painted structure strive to be typical, clear, and correctly reflect the morphology of the structures in each part and adjacent relationship.

3. When drawing, gently draw the outline of the structure with a soft pencil (HB pencil), draw the whole picture with a hard pencil with uniform lines after revision determination; the lines should be continuous and uniform and unrepeatable; the cell structure are represented by dots of uniform size and varying density, without paint shadows and processing with other art modalities.

4. The name and magnification of the drawing are marked at the bottom of the diagram. Draw parallel lines to the right from each of the main structures on the figure, and mark the structure name at the end of the parallel line. If it is not convenient to elicit a parallel line, a slash may be elicited first; then, a parallel line was elicited at the end of the slash. Oblique leads can not cross each other, and the ends of each parallel line should be aligned.

5. All the words marked in picture must be written with pencil clearly.

Experiment 20　Cytochemistry

Cytochemistry is the experimental study of cell biology based on maintaining the original morphological structure of the cell, using chemical reagents to react with intracellular substances, to form a colored precipitate locally in the cell, which reveals intracellular biomacromolecules (such as nucleic acids, proteins, enzymes, etc.), and by microscopic observation, qualitative, localized, and quantitative studies of intracellular biomacromolecules. Cytochemistry is one of the standard methods to study the components of cells.

Section 1　Cytochemistry of Nucleic Acid

【Purpose and requirements】

1. To understand the principle of the Brachet reaction.

2. To master the cytochemical staining methods of DNA and RNA in cells.

【Experimental principle】

Methyl green (MG) and pyronin (P) are alkaline dyes with a positive charge that can be visualized by combining with nucleic acid molecules with negative charge to produce color. In 1940, Brachet revealed Mg-P staining's histochemical basis, so this staining method is also known as the Brachet reaction. The effects of methyl green and pylons are selective. Methyl green has two positive charges, has a strong affinity for double-stranded DNA with a high degree of polymerization, and is consistent with the distance of negatively charged groups on the double helix structure of DNA molecules and easy to bind, so methyl green can make DNA distributed in the nucleus dyed blue or green. The pyronin molecule, which has a positive charge, can only binds single-stranded RNA

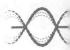

molecules with a low degree of polymerization, staining the RNA in the cytoplasm and nucleoli red.

This indicates that the chromogenic reaction of methyl green and pyronin on nucleic acid is not a chemical action but is related to the degree of DNA and RNA polymerization. DNA, when depolymerized to a certain extent, can also combine with pyronin and appear red. Cells were treated with methyl green-pyronin mixture, in which DNA and RNA show different chromogenic responses, so that DNA and RNA can be analyzed qualitatively, localized, and quantified.

【Experimental supplies】

1. Materials and reagents　Toad, methyl green-pyronin dye, acetone, acetone and xylene (1 : 2) mixture, 70% ethanol, xylene, distilled water.

2. Equipments　Anatomy equipment, microscope, slide, absorbent paper, crayon, coverslip.

【Experimental procedures】

1. Sampling and preparation　See experiment 2 for preparation of toad blood smear.

2. Fixation　Put one blood smear into 70% ethanol, fix it for 5~10min, and then dry it after removing.

3. Dyeing　Draw lines on both ends of the blood film on the blood smear with a crayon to frame the staining site. Add several drops of methyl green-pyronin dye to the surface of the blood smear, and dye for 30min (note: the dye should be given slightly more than necessary, to prevent the surface exposure of the blood smear due to volatilization of the dye during the dyeing).

4. Rinsing　Discard the dye on the blood smear, rinse with distilled water 2~3 times, and blot the water on the back of the slide with absorbent paper, but do not blot the water on the blood film.

5. Color separation and transparency　Put the blood smear into pure acetone for color separation of 2~3s (no more than 10s, otherwise the color will recede), acetone and xylene mixture (1 : 2) for 5s, and xylene for 5min.

6. Microscopic examination　After the images were found on low power objective and high power objective, viewing with an oil immersion objective the cytoplasm is stained red and the nucleus blue-green, whereas its nucleoli are stained red.

【Analysis and thinking】

1. Briefly describe the principle of the Brachet reaction to display DNA and RNA.

2. Why can the cytoplasm and nucleus of toad erythrocyte be stained into different colors by methyl green-pyronin dye?

3. In the Brachet reaction, what color are the nucleoplasm and cytoplasm respectively stained? If the nucleoli are visible, what color should the nucleoli be dyed? What does this difference in dyeing tell us?

4. In which parts of the cell are intracellular DNA and RNA distributed?

【Experimental report】

1. Draw the red blood cell map of the toad with Brachet reaction, and indicate the color of cytoplasm and nucleus, respectively. According to the experimental results, explaining the color differences of nucleus and cytoplasm between treated and untreated specimen.

2. Drawing the distribution of DNA and RNA in toad erythrocytes.

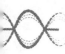

Section 2　Cytochemistry of Protein

【Purpose and requirements】

1. To understand the cytochemical reaction principle of protein.

2. To master the cytochemical staining methods of acidic protein and basic protein in cells.

【Experimental principle】

1. Since the number of basic groups (amino groups) and acidic groups (carboxyl groups) carried in different protein molecules varies, the whole protein is differently positively or negatively charged in different pH solutions. Under physiological conditions, the whole protein with negative charge is acidic protein, and the whole protein with positive charge is basic protein. Therefore, after the nucleic acid was extracted from the sample by trichloroacetic acid treatment, the acid protein and basic protein in the cell could be displayed respectively by staining with different pH solid green dye.

2. Cytoskeleton is a network structure composed of protein fibers in eukaryotic cells, consisting of microfilaments, microtubules, and intermediate filaments. It plays an essential role in cell morphology maintenance, cell growth, movement, division, differentiation, and material transportation. The method of observing cytoskeleton structure with optical microscope is as follows, first, the cells were treated with non-ionic detergent TritonX-100 (polyethylene glycol octyl phenyl ether) to dissolve the plasma membrane, cell wall, 95% of the soluble protein in the cell, and total lipid, but the cytoskeletal protein is preserved without dissolution and destruction. Then, the cytoskeleton structure could be observed clearly under the optical microscope by fixing and non-specific proteins dye coomassie brilliant blue R250 staining.

Under the experimental conditions, the microtubule structure was unstable, while the intermediate filaments around 10nm in diameter were too thin to be distinguished under the optical microscope. Therefore, the cytoskeleton seen under the optical microscope was a bundle of microfilaments formed by multiple microfilaments, called stress fibers.

【Experimental supplies】

1. Materials and reagents　Toad, onion bulbs, human oral mucosal epithelial cells, 5% trichloroacetic acid, 10% formaldehyde, 0.1% acidic solid green dye (pH 2.0), 0.1% alkaline solid green dye (pH 8.0), 6 mmol/L PBS (pH 6.5), disodium hydrogen phosphate citrate buffer (pH 2.2), phosphate buffer (pH 7.2), disodium hydrogen phosphate citrate buffer (pH 8.0), the M-buffer (pH 7.2), 1% TritonX-100, 0.2% coomassie brilliant blue R250 dye, 3% glutaraldehyde, 70% ethanol, normal saline, distilled water.

2. Equipments　Constant temperature water bath, centrifuge, electric furnace, microscope, anatomy equipment, small beaker, slide, coverslip, absorbent paper, dyeing tank, crayon, Petri dish, pipette, toothpick.

【Experimental procedures】

1. Acidic protein and basic protein

1.1　Animal cells

1.1.1　Sampling and preparation: For toad blood smear preparation, see Experiment 2 (or take two toad blood smears that had been prepared).

1.1.2　Fixation: The smear was fixed in 70% ethanol for 5min, then dried at room temperature.

1.1.3　Trichloroacetic acid treating: Put the smear into 60℃ 5% trichloroacetic acid treatment for 30min, Extract to remove nucleic acid. Remove the smear and rinse with running water for more than 3min until there is no trace of trichloroacetic acid on the specimen. Note: Trichloroacetic acid residue can interfere with the staining of solid green dye and affect the observation.

1.1.4　Dyeing: Blot the water on the slide with absorbent paper, and frame out the dyeing part with crayon. The smear intended to show acidic protein was stained with 0.1% acid solid green dye (pH 2.0) for 5~10min, the smear intended to show basic protein was stained with 0.1% alkaline solid green dye (pH 8.0) for 30~60min. The two stained slides were then washed in tap water, and dried at room temperature.

1.1.5　Microscopic examination: After finding the object image on low power objective, use high power objective for observation. At high power objective, the cytoplasm and nucleoli of the samples stained with acidic solid green dye are stained green, indicating the distribution of acidic protein in the cells. In the samples stained with alkaline solid green solution, only the nucleus is stained green. This is the location of basic protein, the histones involved in chromosomes' composition, in the nucleus, while the cytoplasm is colorless.

1.2　Plant cells

1.2.1　Sampling and fixation: Several slices of onion bulb epidermis were taken and placed in a petri dish containing 10% formaldehyde and fixed for 15min. Take out the specimen, put it into a small beaker containing distilled water, draw distilled water with a pipette, rinse the specimen repeatedly, and then suck and discard the distilled water. This step is repeated three times.

1.2.2　Trichloroacetic acid treating: Inject 30ml of 5% trichloroacetic acid into the beaker containing the specimen for full soaking, and then heat the beaker on the electric furnace to keep the temperature of the solution in the beaker at 90℃ for 15min. The treatment solution was discarded, and the specimen was rinsed repeatedly with tap water until the odor of trichloroacetic acid was free.

1.2.3　Dyeing: Half of the specimens were transferred to another beaker, and the specimens in the two beakers were stained for 1~5min with 20ml 0.1% acidic solid green dye (pH 2.0) and 20ml 0.1% alkaline solid green dye (pH 8.0), respectively. Then suck and discard the dye, suck 20ml of pH 2.2 and 20ml of pH 8.0 phosphoric acid buffer with a glue head pipette, and blow and wash for 30s.

Take out the specimens inside two beakers, put them on the slides, and add a drop of the phosphoric acid buffer of pH 2.2 and 8.0, respectively, flatten them with a dissecting needle, and cover the coverslip.

1.2.4　Microscopic examination: The sample stained with 0.1% acidic solid green dye (pH 2.0), whose acidic proteins are stained green; the sample stained with 0.1% alkaline solid green dye (pH 8.0), whose alkaline proteins are stained green. Please compare the intracellular distribution of acidic protein and basic protein based on the observation that the specimens were stained with both stains.

2. Cytoskeleton protein

2.1　Onion epidermal cells

2.1.1　Sampling: Cut onion bulb, avulse the inner epidermis of the middle scale, and cut it

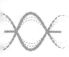

into pieces about 2~3mm^2 in size. The small pieces were dipped into a small beaker containing 5ml 6mmol/L PBS (pH 6.5), treated for 5~10min, and made to sink.

2.1.2   Extraction: PBS was absorbed and discarded, 3ml 1% TritonX-100 was added, processed in a 37℃ incubator for 20~30min, and proteins other than cytoskeleton were extracted.

2.1.3   Washing: 1% TritonX-100 was absorbed and then gently washed with 3ml M-buffer 3 times, 5min each time, to stabilize the cytoskeleton.

2.1.4   Fixing: absorb and discard M-buffer, add 5ml 3% glutaraldehyde, and fix for 15~20min.

2.1.5   Washing: Absorb and discard the fixing solution, and wash with 5ml 6mmol/L PBS (pH 6.5) 3 times, 5min each time. Finally, the absorbent paper is used to absorb the residual liquid.

2.1.6   Dyeing: Add five drops of 0.2% coomassie brilliant blue R250 dye and stain for 3~5min.

2.1.7   Preparation: Absorb and discard the dye, wash it with distilled water 2~3 times, take out the specimen and lay it on the slide, and cover the coverslip on the specimen.

2.1.8   Microscopic examination: The outline of onion epidermal cells can be seen under optical microscope, and there are fiber network structures stained blue and differed in diamete, namely the microfilament bundles of the cytoskeleton. In Some cells, some radially distributed filaments can also be seen at the periphery of the nucleus. The better stained cells are selected, and high power objective is converted, so that the stereoscopic structure of the cytoskeleton could be observed.

2.2   Human oral mucosal epithelial cells

2.2.1   preparation of smear: Scrape human oral mucosal epithelial cells with a clean toothpick, place them in a tube with normal saline, wash and centrifuge for 1~2 times, leaving about 0.5ml of pellet; blow it evenly by pipette to make a cell suspension; then drop the cell suspension to the slide, and smears are prepared and left to dry in the air.

2.2.2   Rinsing: Rinse the dried smear with M-buffer for 3 times.

2.2.3   Extracting: The cell smear was placed in a stained glass tank containing 1% Triton X-100 and treated at room temperature or 37℃ for 20~30min.

2.2.4   Rinsing: Remove the smear from Triton X-100 and rinse with M-buffer solution for 3 times, 3min each time.

2.2.5   Fixation: Use absorbent paper to absorb the excess M-buffer on the smear, put the smear into a glass dyeing tank containing 3% glutaraldehyde, and fix it for 10~15min.

2.2.6   Washing: Take out the smear, absorb the excess fixed solution with absorbent paper, and then wash with phosphate buffer (pH 7.2) for 3 times, 3min each time; finally, the absorbent paper is used to absorb the residual solution.

2.2.7   Dyeing: Add five drops of 0.2% coomassie brilliant blue R250 dye to the smear and stain for 30~60min. Absorb and discard the solution and rinse with distilled water several times carefully.

2.2.8   Microscopic examination: The smear specimen is covered with a coverslip, and then the smear is observed at the microscope. At low power objective, the stress fibers composed of microfilaments in the cytoplasm were purplish-blue and distributed parallel or crossed along the cell's long axis. The nucleus is round and pale blue near the cell's center, with 2~5 dark blue nucleoli in the nucleus. Cells with typical structures were selected for further observation at high power objective.

【Analysis and thinking 】

1. What are the principles that show the acid-base properties of proteins in cells?

2. What is the principle of acidic protein and basic protein staining?

3. Please specify what substance might the colored basic protein be.

4. Why is the pH of solid green dye differently in the experiment displaying acidic protein and basic protein in cells?

【Experimental report 】

1. Drawing the distribution of acidic protein and basic protein in toad erythrocyte.

2. Drawing the cytoskeleton distribution of onion epidermal cells and human oral mucosal epithelial cells.

Section 3　Cytochemistry of carbohydrate

【Purpose and requirements 】

1. Be familiar with the cytochemical reaction principle of polysaccharides.

2. To master the cytochemical staining method of polysaccharides in cells.

【Experimental principle 】

The cytochemistry of carbohydrate is a cytochemical staining method that shows the existence and distribution of polysaccharides in cells, by using the principle of chromogenic reaction of polysaccharides.

1. Periodic acid-Schiff reaction　Monosaccharides in carbohydrate are extracted in the process of histochemical operation such as tissue specimen fixation, dehydration, and embedding. Therefore, polysaccharides, including glycogen, neutral mucopolysaccharides, glycoproteins, and glycolipids, are the main sugars displayed on histochemical specimens. Most of the carbohydrate that animals take into their bodies are converted to fat and stored in adipose tissue, with only a small amount stored in the form of glycogen, which can be quickly broken down when glucose is needed. Glycogen is a polymer of glucose molecules linked together by glycosidic bonds, known as "animal starch", stored mainly in muscle cells and liver cells.

McManus developed periodic acid-Schiff reaction (PAS) in 1946 based on Feulgen reaction, and it is the most classical and direct cytochemical method to show glycogen and other polysaccharides. In this reaction, the glycol group (CHOH-CHOH) of glucose in polysaccharides is oxidized to two aldehyde groups (-CHO) by the strong oxidant periodate, and then the aldehyde group reacts with the Schiff reagent to form insoluble purplish-red complex, which adheres to the site where the polysaccharide exists. The color of the complex is proportional to the content of the polysaccharide.

2. Colour reaction of starch　Starch is a kind of polysaccharide stored in plant cells. It turns blue in iodine solution, when heated, the blue disappears. After cooling, the blue reappears. Starch can be divided into amylose and amylopectin. The blue substance is the unstable iodized starch formed when amylose encounters iodine.

【Experimental supplies】

1. Materials and reagents   Paraffin section of mouse liver, fresh potato, 1% iodine solution

2. Equipments   Microscope, slide, coverslip, tweezers, double-sided blade, absorbent paper, petri dish, writing brush, etc.

【Experimental procedures】

1. PAS reaction   Observing of liver tissue sections of mice stained with PAS: Liver tissue sections of mice stained with PAS were observed under the optical microscope, and showed that hepatocytes appeared slightly polygonal in shape, with one or two nuclei stained blue in the center, and many purplish-red glycogen particles could be seen in the cytoplasm (Fig.20-1). The glycogen granules in liver cells were different in number and size, some of them were fine granules, and others were large ones. The glycogen granules in the peripheral hepatocytes in the section tend to be on one side of the cell (opposite the boundary) in a half-moon-shape so that the distribution of glycogen in peripheral hepatocytes was wavy. This is caused by the penetration of the stationary solution to push the glycogen particles to one side of the cells during the preparation process, and does not represent the distribution of glycogen in the cells under living conditions. Besides, unstained vacuoles of varying sizes can be seen between the glycogen granules, which result from fat droplets being dissolved by fat-soluble solvents during the preparation process.

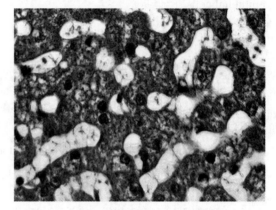

Fig.20-1　PAS stained mouse liver tissue (glycogen granules in hepatocytes showed)

2. Starch chromogenic reaction

2.1　Slice with free hands

2.1.1   Potatoes were cut into small segments of approximately 0.5cm × 0.5cm × 3cm and the cut surface was pared so as to freehand slice. Take a petri dish and prepare water.

2.1.2   With the thumb and index finger of the left hand, clamp the potato strip so that it is fixed; to prevent knife wounds, the thumb should be slightly lower than the index finger, and make the top of the potato beyond the index finger 2~3mm.

2.1.3   Before freehand slicing, dip some water on the knife-edge to play a smooth role. The right broad thumb and index finger pinch the lower right corner of the blade with the knife edge inward and parallel to the potato cut surface.

2.1.4   The left hand remains still, and the right upper arm drives the forearm and the right hand to move, so that the knife edge cuts from the outside in the left front direction to the inside in the right back direction. Cut several slices in succession for later use.

Note: When cutting by hand, use only arm force, not wrist or knuckle force. Hands should not lean on the body or press on the table, and the action should be agile. To cut off at a time, do not stop halfway, do not make "drag-saw" type cutting. During sectioning, the knife-edge and material should be continuously moistened with water to keep the knife-edge sharp and avoid the material's deformation. The key to freehand slicing is to cut thin and evenly.

2.2　Dyeing：Choose a thin and uniform potato chip, move it to the slide, add one drop of 1% iodine solution, it can be seen that it is dyed blue immediately, and then cover the coverslip. The spilled iodine liquid is soaked with absorbent paper.

2.3　Microscopic examination：It can be seen that there are many oval starch grains dyed blue in the polygonal paren-chyma cells (Fig.20-2), and there are clear umbilical and ring lines on the slightly stained starch grains.

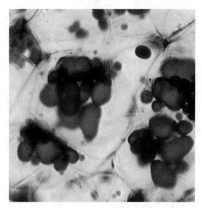

Fig.20-2　Parenchyma cells of potato tubers (starch granules shown)

【 Analysis and thinking 】

1. What are the kinds of sugars in animal and plant cells?　What are the main energy-storing substances?

2. What is the principle of demonstrating glycogen in animal cells?

3. Why was starch that had been exposed to iodine that turned blue, the blue color disappeared upon heating and reappeared upon cooling?

【 Experimental report 】

1. Drawing represents the distribution of glycogen in hepatocytes, and indicating the glycogen granules.

2. Draw 2~3 potato parenchyma cells and mark starch granules and cell walls.

Experiment 21　Microstructure of Cell

【 Purpose and requirements 】

1. Be familiar with the morphology of organelles and their distribution in cells at the optical microscope.

2. Be familiar with the principle and method of supravital staining of mitochondria and vacuoles.

3. To master the distribution of mitochondria and vacuoles in cells at the optical microscope.

【 Experimental principle 】

Supravital staining is an in vitro staining method for living tissues or cells obtained from the body. The dye used for supravital staining is specific, non-toxic, or less toxic, does not affect or less affect cells' life activities, and does not produce any physical and chemical changes to cells and tissues.

1. Mitochondrial supravital staining　Janus Green B, an alkaline dye, is a specific living dye of mitochondria, which is less toxic and fat-soluble. It can pass through the plasma membrane and mitochondrial membrane into the mitochondria and bind to the negatively charged inner membrane and cristal membrane through the positively charged dye groups in its structure. Mitochondria, which contain various enzymes related to energy metabolism, are essential place of energy metabolism in

cells. Among mitochondria, the cytochrome oxidase on the intima and cristal membrane can make the bound Janus green B always maintain the oxidation state and become blue-green (colored state). In contrast, the Janus green B in the cytoplasm around the mitochondria is reduced to a colorless base (colorless state).

2. Vacuolar supravital staining   In animal cells, vacuoles formed by monolayer membrane belongs to the vacuolar system (except mitochondrial membrane and nuclear membrane), including Golgi body, lysosome, endoplasmic reticulum, phagosome, and pinosome. Neutral red, a weakly basic dye, is a specific in vivo dye for vacuoles, which only stains the vacuoles of living cells red, while the nucleus, mitochondria, and cytosol are not stained at all. The staining mechanism of neutral red may be related to the specific proteins in vacuoles. Chondrocytes contain more rough endoplasmic reticulum and well-developed Golgi body, which can synthesize and secrete cartilage mucin and collagen fibers, and well-developed vacuole system. Therefore, cartilage tissue is often used as the material for vacuolar supravital staining.

3. Golgi body silver staining   Golgi body was discovered in 1898 by Italian scientist C Golgi when staining nerve cells with silver staining. Due to the Golgi body's argyrophilic nature, the black or brown silver chromate precipitate formed by the reaction of potassium dichromate and silver nitrate is deposited in neurons.

4. Gentian violet staining of the centrosome   The pericentriolar material around the centrosome acts as the microtubule organizing center. The γ-tubulin ring complex (γ-TuBC) in the microtubule organizing center is like a seed, which can combine with the α/β tubulin heterodimer, that is, it has nucleation, from which the microtubule grows and lengthens. When the chromosomes in the M phase were stained with basic dye gentian violet, the cells' centrosome could be clearly seen.

【Experimental supplies】

1. Materials and reagents   rabbit, toad, mouse kidney section, rabbit spinal ganglion silver staining section, gentian violet stained section of the uterus of equine roundworm, 1/300 Janus Green B solution (for rabbits and amphibians), 0.80%Ringer solution (for rabbits), 0.65%Ringer solution (for amphibians), and 1/3 000 neutral red solution (for amphibians).

2. Equipments   anatomical equipment, anatomical plates, Petri dish, slide, coverslip, pipette, absorbent paper, syringe (for killing rabbits), microscope, lens paper, cedar (or liquid paraffin), anhydrous ethanol (or ethyl ether ethanol mixture).

【Experimental procedures】

1. Observing of microstructure section of cell

1.1   Mitochondria (mouse kidney section): At low power objective many circular and oval structures can be seen, this is the transverse section of the renal tubules. On transverse section, the renal tubule is composed of a layer of tightly packed epithelial cells. The cells are tapered, but the cells' outline is not clear. Further observation by high power objective or oil immersion objective showed that there were many short rod-shaped or granular structures stained blue-black in the cytoplasm of renal tubular epithelial cells, namely mitochondria. In general, there are more mitochondria in the cytoplasm at the base of the cell (Fig.21-1).

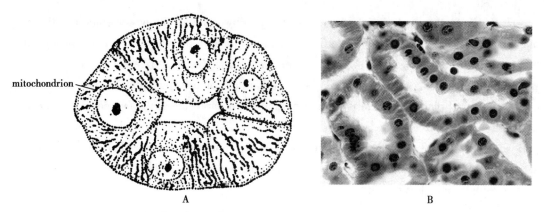

Fig.21-1 Mitochondria in renal tubular cells

A. Pattern diagram;B. Microstructure diagram.

1.2 Golgi body (rabbit spinal ganglion section):At low power objective,the brown nerve fiber bundles separate the ganglion cells (oval or round) into groups;at high power objective, it can be seen that the central staining of ganglion cells is pale yellow or vacuolated,where the nucleus is located. In some ganglion cells,yellowish-brown,highly refractive nucleoli can be seen in the nuclear center. The cytoplasm around the nucleus is dyed light yellow,in which there are curved linear,reticular,and granular structures dyed black or brown,that is,Golgi bodies (Fig.21-2).

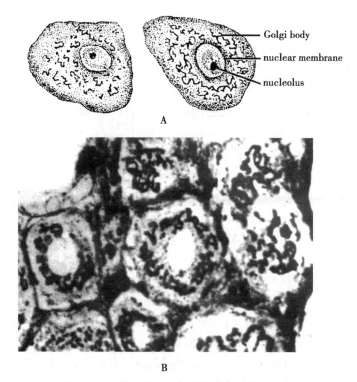

Fig.21-2 Golgi body in spinal ganglion cells

A. Pattern diagram ;B. Microstructure diagram.

1.3 Centrosome (uterine section of equine roundworm): At low power objective, there are many large cavities surrounded by a fertilized egg membrane in the uterine cavity of Ascaris equi, that is, the surrounding egg cavity, in which there are fertilized eggs at different phases of M phase. In the fertilized eggs at metaphase, it can be seen that dark blue striped chromosomes are arranged on the equatorial plate, and there is a small particle dyed dark blue at the two poles of the cell on both sides of the chromosomes, which is called centriole. The centriole and the surrounding dense pericentriolar material are called the centrosome. At high power objective, radial stellar rays can be seen around the centrosome, and spindles composed of many microtubules can be observed between the two centrosomes (Fig.21-3).

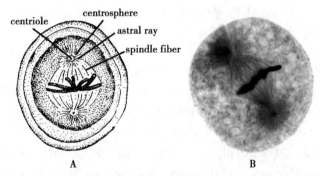

Fig.21-3 The mitotic metaphase of fertilized egg of Ascaris equi (centrosome shown)

A. Pattern diagram; B. Microstructure diagram.

2. Supravital staining

2.1 Mitochondrial supravital staining

2.1.1 Sampling and dyeing: The rabbit are sacrificed by air embolism method. The abdominal surface of rabbit are placed upward in an anatomical plate, and the abdominal cavity is quickly opened. A small piece of liver tissue (2~5mm^3) is dissected at the edge of the rabbit liver and placed in a petri dish containing 0.80% Ringer's solution. Gently squeeze the liver tissue with tweezers, wash away the blood, then clip the liver tissue with tweezers and place it on the slide, and add a few drops of 1/300 Janus green B solution to the liver tissue so that the lower part of the tissue mass is immersed in the solution and the upper part is exposed outside the solution. The cytochrome oxidase in the cell can be fully oxidized (mitochondrial staining) under aerobic conditions until the tissue mass' edge is dyed blue-green. It is usually necessary to dye 30min.

Toad liver can also be used in this experiment; the difference is that 0.65% Ringer's solution is used to wash away blood of toad liver, the staining method and staining time are the same as above.

2.1.2 Preparation: After staining, the tissue block was minced first with scissors; then tweezers were used to press the tissue block, at which point some cells or cell clusters would be detached from the tissue block; remove the slightly larger tissue mass, leave the separated cells or cell clusters on the slide, add a drop of 0.80% Ringer's solution (for rabbit liver) or 0.65% Ringer's solution (for toad liver) to the slides; finally cover with a coverslip, and absorb the excess solution.

2.1.3 Microscopic examination: at the optical microscope, it can be seen that some short rod-shaped or round granular structures dyed blue green, i.e., mitochondria, are scattered around the nucleus of rabbit hepatocytes. The mitochondria in toad hepatocytes are granular and stained blue-green with a more peripheral distribution of nuclei.

2.2　Vacuolar supravital staining

2.2.1　Sampling: One toad are sacrificed by disrupting the brain and spinal cord, the thoracoabdominal cavity is cut, the xiphoid process is exposed, and a small piece is cut at the edge of the xiphoid cartilage and placed on the slide.

2.2.2　Dyeing: Drop 2 drops 1/3 000 neutral red solution on the specimen of the slide. The solution is removed by blotting with absorbent paper 15 min after staining, add one drop of 0.65% Ringer's solution, cover with a coverslip, and blot off the excess Ringer's solution.

2.2.3　Microscopic examination: On optical microscope, it can be seen that the chondrocytes are oval, and there are many vesicles in the cytoplasm that stain rose red and vary in size, that is, the vacuole system of chondrocytes.

【 Analysis and thinking 】

1. What is the principle of supravital staining of mitochondria and vacuoles?

2. Please briefly describe microstructure characteristics of mitochondria and Golgi body.

3. Please briefly describe microstructure characteristics of rabbit (or toad) hepatocytes and toad xiphoid chondrocytes supravital staining.

4. When observing silver stained sections of rabbit spinal ganglion, Why are there no nucleoli in some ganglion nuclei?

【 Experimental report 】

1. Drawing structural map of rat renal tubular cells.

2. Drawing structural map of rabbit spinal ganglion cells.

3. Drawing structural map of toad hepatocyte with mitochondrial supravital staining.

Experiment 22　Physiological Activity of Cell

【 Purpose requirements 】

1. To understand the structural characteristics of cilia and flagella, and the modes of their movements.

2. To understand the general rules of the plasma membrane permeability, the relationship between hemolysis and permeability of plasma membrane.

3. To understand the selective permeability of the plasma membrane and the mechanism of hemolysis by observing the hemolysis phenomenon of animal red blood cells' in different solutions.

【 Experimental principle 】

The cells' physiological activities contain cell movement, material transport from the plasma membrane, intracellular material metabolism, energy metabolism, cell proliferation and differentiation, cell response to the external environment, muscle cell contraction, the conduction of nerve cell excitation, and so on. In this experiment, through the observation of cell movement and plasma membrane permeability, we have a preliminary understanding of cell physiological activities.

1. Cell movement　Cilia and flagella are rod-shaped structures with motile function projecting from the cell surface of unicellular and multicellular organisms. Usually, the multiple, short ones are called cilia, and the few and long ones are called flagella, which all push the cells forward. Cilia and flagella are composed of axoneme lined by longitudinally arranged microtubule bundles and the plasma membrane on the outer side; The longitudinal direction consists of two parts, the basal body, which is buried inside the cell, and the rod portion, which protrudes to the cell surface. The microtubule constitution differs in each segment axoneme of cilia and flagella, with microtubules of the middle axoneme showing a "$9 \times 2+2$" configuration: nine sets of doublet microtubules (tube A and tube B) and two central microtubules. The doublet disassembles ATP molecules by the A-tubule dynein arm (ATPase), releasing energy to generate sliding between the doublets; sliding is converted into bending by the attachment of doublets to the central microtubule radial filaments, causing the movement of cilia and flagella.

The synergistic wobble of the cilia of the mucosal epithelial cells of the toads' respiratory tract can promote the passage of fluid and solid particles through its surface. The structure of the sperm tail is similar to that of cilia and flagella. The distal centrosome far from the nucleus of spermatid evolves into the axoneme of the sperm, and the axoneme is also a "$9 \times 2+2$" structure, which is the motor organ of the sperm.

2. Permeability of plasma membrane　Plasma membrane is a kind of semi-permeable membrane, which is selective to substances' permeability. When the red blood cells are placed in the hypotonic solution, because the osmotic pressure is higher inside the cell than outside, the water molecules quickly enter the cell, causing the cell to burst, hemolysis occurs, and the turbid red blood cell suspension will turn into a red and transparent hemoglobin solution. When red blood cells are placed in isotonic solutions of different solutes, the permeability of erythrocyte plasma membrane to various solute molecules is different, resulting in the different speed of solute molecules penetrating into the cells, as a result, hemolysis time caused by increased osmotic pressure, water intake, and plasma membrane rupture is also different. The plasma membrane's permeability to the substance is related to the molecular weight, lipid solubility, and whether it is charged or not. Accordingly, the permeability of the plasma membrane to various substances can be estimated by measuring hemolysis time.

【Experimental supplies】

1. Materials and reagents　Male toad, rabbit, 0.17mol/L Sodium Chloride, 0.17mol/L ammonium Chloride, 0.17mol/L ammonium Acetate, 0.17mol/L Sodium nitrate, 0.12mol/L ammonium oxalate, 0.12mol/L Sodium Sulfate, 0.32mol/L glucose, 0.32mol/L Glycerin, 0.32mol/L ethanol, 0.32mol/L Propanol, 0.27mol/L Sodium Chloride, aseptic Heparin (500U/ml) normal saline, distilled water.

2. Equipments　Microscope, cedar oil (or liquid paraffin), anhydrous ethanol (or ether ethanol mixture), lens paper, anatomical equipment, ophthalmic scissors, wax tray, pin, toothpick, slide, coverslip, petri dish, pipette, absorbent paper, wax chips, beaker, test tube, test tube holder, 50ml syringe, 5ml syringe, sulfuric acid paper.

【 Experimental procedures 】

1. Cilia movement of epithelial cells in maxillary mucosa of toad

1.1　One male toad was sacrificed by disrupting the brain and spinal cord; the toad's abdomen is up, its limbs were unfolded, and a pin was used to anchor it to a wax tray.

1.2　Cut backward about 1cm along the two sides mouth angle of the toad, overturn its jaw and fix it on the abdomen to expose the pharynx (Fig.22-1).

1.3　The wax chips were placed in the midline of maxilla, which is 1cm from the larynx and observe whether the wax shavings move or not, and the direction of movement. Think about why the wax particles move, and record how long it takes for the wax particles to move until they disappear.

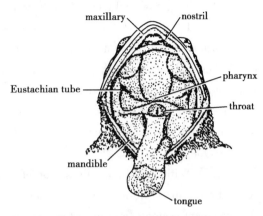

Fig.22-1　Internal surface of toad buccal cavity

1.4　A small mucosa piece about 2mm × 2mm in the anterior part of the maxillary larynx was snipped with ophthalmic scissors, picked up the mucosal blocks with a toothpick, and attach the vertical section to the slide. Add one drop of saline to the specimen and cover the coverslip.

1.5　Microscopic examination: Find the site where the cilia motility at low power objective first and then, change to the high power objective to carefully observe the movement pattern of the cilia.

2. Flagellum movement of toad sperm

2.1　The sacrificed male toad was cut open to the thoracoabdominal wall along the abdomen's midline to expose the yellow cylinder shaped seminal nests.

2.2　Snip the seminal nests into a petri dish filled with saline, swing one end in water by holding it with tweezers, and wash away blood.

2.3　Move the washed seminal nests into a clean petri dish, mince it well with ophthalmic scissors, and add a few drops of normal saline to mix.

2.4　Aspirate the liquid from the petri dish with a pipette, place one drop onto a slide, cover a coverslip, and examine microscopically 2~3min later.

2.5　Microscopic examination: Looking at it with low power objective (dimming the light), you can see that there are many moving sperm in the field of vision. Choose slow-moving sperm and observe them with high power objective or oil immersion objective. Toad sperm consists of head, neck, and tail. The head is long conical shape, the neck is very short (with anterior and posterior centrosomes, not easy to see), the tail is slender, and sometimes wavy margins are seen, consisting mainly of axonemes whose structure resembles a flagellum. The sperm moves by bending and swinging the tail.

3. Permeability of plasma membrane

3.1　Preparation of a 10% rabbit red blood cell suspension: Normal saline 45ml was added in the beaker beforehand. A rabbit was sacrificed by air embolism method, and the thoracic cavity

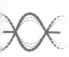

of the rabbit was cut to expose the heart; a 500U/ml sterile heparin 0.5ml moist syringe barrel was drawn, and the blood in the rabbit heart was drawn to 5ml, injected into a beaker, shaken gently, mixed, and prepared as a 10% rabbit red blood cell suspension. Rabbit erythrocyte suspensions appear as red opaque fluid in appearance.

3.2　Changes of erythrocytes in different osmotic solutions

3.2.1　Each group (2 persons) takes 3 test tubes, which were numbered as No.1 (hypotonic), No.2 (isotonic) and No.3 (hypertonic). First, add 0.3ml of 10% RBC suspension into three test tubes, then add 3ml of distilled water, 0.17mol/L sodium chloride and 0.27mol/L sodium chloride solution into test tubes 1, 2 and 3 respectively, finally seal the tube orifice with sulfuric acid paper and invert it once. The hemolysis of erythrocytes (color change of solution, transparency of solution, etc.) in hypotonic, isotonic, and hyperosmotic solutions was observed separately, and the results were recorded.

3.2.2　With a toothpick dip a drop of each of the above No.1 (hypotonic), No.2 (isotonic), No.3 (hypertonic) solutions at a slide separately, then cover a coverslip. Rabbit erythrocytes in the hypotonic, isotonic, and hypertonic solutions were examined on high power objective for any differences in morphology.

3.3　Determination of the permeability of various substances to the plasma membrane of erythrocytes: Take 10 tubes, numbered sequentially. 2ml of the prepared 10 kinds of isotonic solution was added to each tube, and then 0.2ml of 10% rabbit red blood cell suspension was added to each tube, respectively, gently shaking and mixing. The hypotonic dissolving tube was used as a control to observe the color change of each tube solution, and the hemolysis time was recorded to analyze the reason why different solutions caused difference of hemolysis time.

3.4　Judgment criteria for hemolysis

3.4.1　Non-hemolysis: The liquid is divided into two layers, the upper layer is light yellow and transparent, and the lower layer is red and opaque.

3.4.2　Incomplete hemolysis: The solution is turbid, and the upper layer turns red.

3.4.3　Complete hemolysis: The solution turns red and transparent.

【 Analysis and thinking 】

1. What are the structure and movement mechanisms of flagella and cilia?

2. Why can the wax chips move in the ciliary motility experiment on the epithelial cells of the toad maxillary mucosa? How do they move? How long does it take for the wax chips move from start to disappearance?

3. Please illustrate the effect of lipid solubility on plasma membrane permeability based on experimental results.

4. What is the difference in hemolysis time of red blood cells in different solutions? Why?

【 Experimental report 】

1. Drawing rabbit red blood cell morphologies in isotonic and hypertonic solution states were plotted separately.

2. Please list a table that indicates the results of rabbit erythrocyte permeability experiments and analyze them.

Experiment 23　Ultrastructure of Cell

【Purpose and requirements】

By viewing video materials and observing electron microscope (EM) photographs, master various organelles' ultrastructure characteristics and deepen your understanding of related theoretical knowledge and the relationship between cell ultrastructure and function.

【Experimental principle】

Ultrastructure, also known as submicroscopic structure, refers to the collective term for cell structures beyond an optical microscope's resolution level that can only be observed by an electron microscope. The resolution of electron microscopy is much higher than that of optical microscopy. It can distinguish various organelles, cell surface structure, various cell junctions, as well as various pathogenic microorganisms such as bacteria(including nanobacteria), mycoplasma and viruses.

According to the structure and use, electron microscope can be divided into transmission electron microscopy, scanning electron microscopy, reflectance electron microscopy and emission electron microscopy. Among them, transmission electron microscopy (TEM) and scanning electron microscopy (SEM) are most commonly used. Transmission electron microscopy is commonly used to observe the fine structures that cannot be resolved by common optical microscope, and scanning electron microscopy is mainly used to observe the morphology of the specimen surface.

【Experimental supplies】

Video data, EM photographs.

【Experimental procedures】

1. Playing video data of cellular ultrastructure.

2. Observing the EM photographs of the cellular ultrastructure and identify ultrastructure of each part of the cell.

【Summary】

1. Plasma membrane　On the EM photographs of the plasma membrane of human RBC, it can be seen that the plasma membrane at the outermost edge of the cell has a three-layer structure. The inner and outer layers are dense layers with higher electron density (dark color), and the area between the two layers are loose layers (light color) with lower electron density, whose total thickness is 7.5~10nm (Fig.23-1). In addition to the plasma membrane, organelles' limiting membrane also has this three-layer structure called the unit membrane.

2. Nucleus　The nucleus is mostly located in the center of the cell (Fig.23-2) and includes several parts of the nuclear envelope, chromatin, nucleolus, and nuclear matrix.

2.1　Nuclear envelope: For the electron microscope, the nuclear envelope comprises two unit membranes (the inner nuclear membrane and the outer nuclear membrane) and the perinuclear space between them. Note: do not mistake this structure for the three layered structure of the unit membrane. There are granular ribosomal attachments to the outer surface of the outer nuclear membrane, which is connected to the endoplasmic reticulum. The perinuclear space communicates

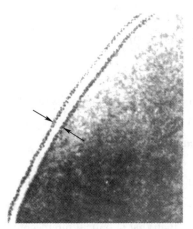

Fig.23-1　Ultrastructure of the
plasma membrane

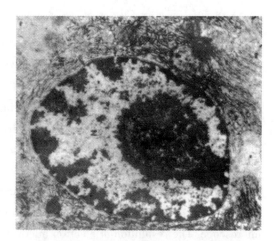

Fig.23-2　Ultrastructure of the nucleus

with the lumen of the endoplasmic reticulum. The inner and outer nuclear membranes fuse to form evenly distributed nuclear pores, which are channels for material exchange between the nucleus and the cytoplasm.

Observe the structure of the lipid bilayer cross-sections of the nuclear envelope shown by the EM photographs of amphibian intestinal epithelial cells and embryonic mesenchymal cells freeze fracture etching replica.

2.2　Chromatin: Chromatin is a substance within the nucleus of interphase cells that can be colored by basic dyes and is divided into two categories based on its morphology and function: euchromatin and heterochromatin. The granular or block structures with deeply tinting, and variable morphology and size is heterochromatin. Between heterochromatin, lighter, loose, fine granular or filamentous structures are euchromatin.

Observe the chromatin structure revealed by EM photographs of amphibian intestinal epithelial cells and guinea pig plasma cells.

2.3　Nucleolus: On electron microscopy, the nucleolus is a fibrous mesh structure without membrane coating, composed of 3 characteristic areas incompletely separated by fiber center, dense fiber center, and particle component. The fiber center, the site of rRNA gene (rDNA) presence, appears as a patchy lightly stained area of low electron density surrounded by a ring-shaped or semilunar dense fiber component of highest electron density in the nucleolus. The particle component are located on the nucleolus periphery, with a particle diameter of 15-20nm, and contain ribosomal subunit precursor particles at different processing stages. The particle component is the major structure of the nucleolus, and the size of the nucleolus is mainly determined by the particle component. The heterochromatin surrounding the nucleolus is called nucleolus associated chromatin, and the euchromatin that extends into the fibers center within the nucleolus is called nucleolar chromatin.

Observe the structure of the nucleolus in the nucleus revealed by EM photographs of guinea pig acini.

2.4　Nuclear matrix: The nuclear matrix is filled in the chromatin and nucleolar space and is an amorphous substance with low electron density. And the nuclear matrix located in the nucleolus is also called the nucleolar matrix.

3. Endoplasmic reticulum   The endoplasmic reticulum is divided into the rough endoplasmic reticulum and smooth endoplasmic reticulum depending on whether or not ribosomes are attached to the outer surface of the membrane. The rough endoplasmic reticulum is flat sac like, interconnected to form a membranous duct system. On electron microscopy, it can be seen that the membrane is dark, while the cavity is light, and granular ribosomes are attached to the outer surface of the membrane. The smooth endoplasmic reticulum appears as a branching tubule and vesicle, some of them are connected to form a net, the membrane surface is smooth, and no ribosomes are attached (Fig.23-3).

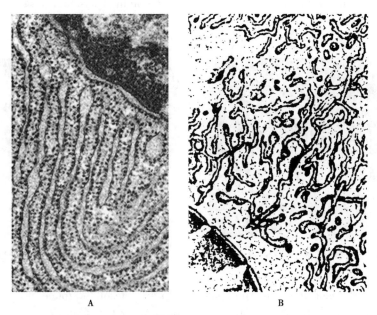

A   B

Fig.23-3   Ultrastructure of the endoplasmic reticulum

A. Rough endoplasmic reticulum; B. Smooth endoplasmic reticulum.

Observe the structure revealed by EM photographs of the rough endoplasmic reticulum in bat membranous acinar cells and mouse liver cells, and the smooth endoplasmic reticulum in human adrenal cortex cells.

4. Golgi body   The Golgi body is formed from vesicle-like structures of different shapes formed by the unit membrane (Fig.23-4), which include flat vesicles, large vesicles, and small vesicles. The flat vesicles is the most prominent part of the Golgi body, usually consist of an overlap of 4-8 layers of flattened vesicles curved into an arch shaped shape with a narrow lumen. The flat vesicles have convex and concave sides: the convex surface, also known as the forming surface, faces the cytoplasm and endoplasmic reticulum; the concave surface, also known as the mature surface (secretion surface), is close to the plasma membrane, and the concave surface can expand into large vesicles. Large vesicles are distributed on the mature surface, migrate from the mature face, and contain secretory granules formed by the progressive concentration of secretory proteins. The small

vesicles of the forming surface are budding from the nearby rough endoplasmic reticulum.

Observe the structure of the Golgi body in EM photographs of spermatogonia and epididymis cells from rat testes.

5. Lysosome　The lysosome is a spherical body enclosed by a single-layer unit membrane containing various acid hydrolases (Fig.23-5). On electron microscopy, the lysosome with uniform electron density for the contents is called the primary lysosome; the lysosome with uneven electron density for the contents is called the secondary lysosome, which is undergoing digestion. Lysosomes are named according to their functional status and the content digested. For example, Residual bodies containing undigested residual material, autophagolysosomes containing mitochondrial remnants are all secondary lysosome. On electron microscopy, attention should be paid to distinguish between lysosomes and mitochondria. There are no cristae in the lysosome, and the electron density is high.

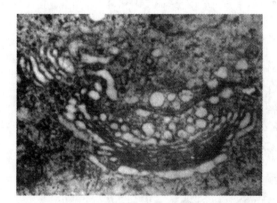
Fig.23-4　Ultrastructure of the Golgi body

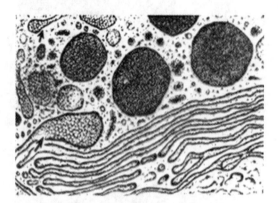
Fig.23-5　Ultrastructure of lysosome

Observe the EM photographs of rat hepatocyte. In the cytosol, the round or oval structure with high electron density and no cristae is the primary lysosome. Observe the polycystic body revealed by the EM photographs of mouse ileum cells.

6. Peroxisome　Peroxisomes are round or elliptical organelles surrounded by a layer of unit membrane. They are generally smaller than lysosomes and contain particulate matter with medium electron density. Observe the peroxisomes in rat and human hepatocytes on electron microscopy, peroxisomes in rat hepatocyte are spherical with low electron density, covered by monolayer membrane, without cristae inside, but with a dark nucleoid inside, which is crystal of urate oxidase. Nucleoids are absent from peroxisomes in human hepatocytes.

Please compare the morphology and structure of peroxisomes with mitochondria and lysosomes.

7. Mitochondria　Mitochondrion is enclosed structure surrounded by a double-layered unit membrane (Fig.23-6). The cavity between the inner and outer membrane is called the intermembrane space (or outer cavity), the inner membrane is folded inward to form plate-like or tubular cristae, and the cavity enclosed by the inner membrane is called the stromal cavity (or inner cavity). The inner membrane, outer membrane, and cristae membrane show dark linear structures. There are many dark spherical bodies (elementary particle) attached to the cristae membrane and

inner membrane. The electron density of the material in the intermembrane space and the stromal cavity is low, and the color is light. The matrix contains electron dense matrix particles. On the negative-stained EM photographs, it can be clearly seen that the white elementary particle on the inner membrane are composed of the ball, the handle, and the base sheet.

8. Ribosome　The ribosome comprises two subunits: a large subunit and a small subunit, without the unit membrane coating. The ribosomes

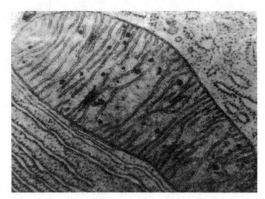

Fig.23-6　Ultrastructure of mitochondrion

attached to the rough endoplasmic reticulum are called attached ribosome, and those free to the cytoplasm are called free ribosome. Multiple ribosomes attach to a chain of mRNA molecules to form a polysome.

On electron microscopy, the ribosome is granular with high electron density and dark color. On the electron microscope photograph of mouse hepatocyte, there are many dark granular structures on the rough endoplasmic reticulum membrane, namely, attached ribosomes.

Polysomes in the cytoplasm are distributed in clusters, appear helical and beaded, and enlarged images of 5-8 or even more ribosomes, which are strings of a linear mRNA molecule, are also seen. On the EM photographs processed by the negative stain technique and at a magnification of $\times 400\,000$, the 80S ribosome appears light in color, and both large and small subunits can be distinguished.

9. Centriole　The centriole, the main constituent of the centrosome, is a cylindrical body. The centrioles that make up the centrosome exist in pairs and are perpendicular to each other. The wall of the cylinder is composed of 9 groups of triplex microtubules arranged in longitudinal rows. On the electron microscopy, the darker tubular structure on the centrioles' longitudinal section is the microtubules that make up the centrioles. On the cross-section, it can be seen that each centriole is composed of nine groups of triplet microtubules, each group of 3 microtubules arranged obliquely, such as the blades of a windmill.

Observe the centrioles that constitute the centrosome on the EM photographs of chicken embryonic membranous gland cells.

10. Microtubule and Microfilament Microtubule is a hollow tubular structure with an outer diameter of 24 to 26nm, dispersed in the cytoplasm. Microfilament is a solid fibrous structure with a 5-6nm diameter, often in bundles arranged in parallel under the plasma membrane, and some are scattered and interwoven into a network (Fig.23-7).

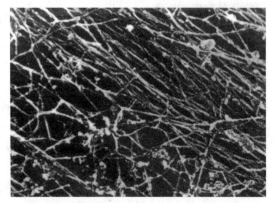

Fig.23-7　Ultrastructure of microtubules and microfilaments

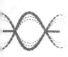

Microtubules and microfilaments in longitudinal sections were observed on the EM photographs of rat glomerulus cells.

11. The whole picture of cells　Observe the EM micrographs of rat hepatocyte.

【Analysis and thinking】

What are the ultrastructure characteristics of various organelles on electron microscope? What are their functions ?

【Experimental report】

Observe the received EM photographs, and mark the ultrastructural name of the indicated part in the "∨" manner on the corresponding position of the table.

Experiment 24　Cell Division

【Purpose and requirements】

1. To master the characteristics of cell morphology and structural changes in each phase of mitosis.

2. Be familiar with the basic process of meiosis and each stage's morphological characteristic.

3. To master the morphological characteristics of chromosomes at each stage of meiotic prophase Ⅰ, metaphase Ⅰ and metaphase Ⅱ.

【Experimental principle】

Cells proliferate by dividing and organisms achieve the purpose of individual growth and reproduction through cell division.

Mitosis is the primary proliferation mode of eukaryotic cells. The morphology of the nucleus changes significantly during cell division. The temporary organelles (mitotic apparatus) specialized in cell division functions can ensure that the two sets of replicated genetic material are equally distributed to the two daughter cells, so this way of cell division is called mitosis. According to the morphological characteristics, the continuous process of mitosis can be divided into four stages: prophase, metaphase, anaphase and telophase.

Meiosis is a unique way of cell division during the formation of germ cells in sexual reproduction individuals, including two consecutive divisions. Since chromosomes are only replicated once before the first meiosis (meiosis Ⅰ) and not replicated before the second meiosis (meiosis Ⅱ), so that the chromosomes of 4 gamete cells produced by meiosis are only half of the number of chromosomes in cells before meiosis, and this way of cell division is called meiosis.

The meiotic process is essentially identical to mitosis and is mainly distinguished by the long duration of prophase (prophase Ⅰ) of meiosis Ⅰ and the complex morphological changes of chromosomes, which is the most characteristic period during meiosis Ⅰ. According to chromosomal morphological characteristics, prophase Ⅰ can be divided into five subphases : leptotene, zygotene, pachytene, diplotene, and diakinesis.

Since locust has few chromosomes, which is easy to observe, operate, and convenient to obtain materials, so it is an ideal material for studying animal cell meiosis. Locust somatic cells, primary oocytes, and primary spermatocytes each have 11 pairs of autosomes. There are two X chromosomes

(XX) in female locust somatic cells and only one X chromosome (X) in male locust somatic cells, so there are 24 chromosomes (2n=22+XX) in female locust somatic cells, while 23 chromosomes (2n=22+X) in male locust somatic cells. In the process of meiosis to generate germ cells, the egg cells formed by female locusts all have 12 chromosomes (n=11+X); the sperm cells formed by male locusts have two types—11 chromosomes (n=11+0) and 12 chromosomes (n=11+X). The two types each account for half.

【Experimental supplies】

1. Materials and reagents　The treated onion root tips, transverse section of the uterus of equine roundworm, tabletting of the male locusts sperm nest, improved phenol fuchsin dye, Carnoy's fixative, 1mol/L HCl solution (60℃ preheated), 95% ethanol, 85% ethanol, 70% ethanol, distilled water.

2. Equipments　Tweezer, slide, coverslip, absorbent paper, microscope, cedar oil (or liquid paraffin), absolute ethanol (or ether-ethanol mixture), lens paper.

【Experimental procedures】

1. Mitosis

1.1　Plant cells

1.1.1　Preparation of onion root tips tabletting:

1.1.1.1　Onion root tip treating: When the root is 2cm long, cut the root tip, immerse it in Carnoy's fixative for 4h, and then store it in 95% and 85% ethanol for 30min, and finally store it in 70% ethanol (complete before the experiment).

1.1.1.2　Hydrolysis: Take out the root tip and place it on a slide, add small volume of 1mol/L HCl solution (60℃) dropwise to the root tip to hydrolyze for 8min, and wash with distilled water three times.

1.1.1.3　Staining and tabletting: Cut the milky white meristem zone of the root tip and mash it gently with tweezers. Add one drop of modified phenol fuchsin staining solution, stain for 20min, and cover a coverslip. After covering the coverslip with a piece of absorbent paper, press it vertically with your thumb; then press one end of the coverslip with one finger first, and tap it lightly with a pencil eraser with the other hand to press the cells into a uniform thin layer (when tapping, do not move the coverslip).

1.1.2　Observing of mitotic specimens of root tip cells: Take the root tip tabletting and find the root tip end on low power objective. From the root tip end up, the root tip is divided into root-crown, growth zone, elongation zone, and root hair zone (Fig.24-1). Select the growth zone at the tip

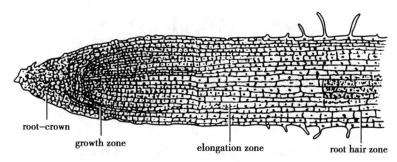

Fig.24-1　Longitudinal section of onion root tip

of the root tip to observe, you can see that the cells are square, deeply stained, and tightly arranged in rows. Please move the specimen slowly, select the part where the cell division is vigorous for observation at high power objective, many cells in different division stages can be seen (Fig.24-2). The structure of each phase of the cell cycle is characterized as follows (Fig.24-3):

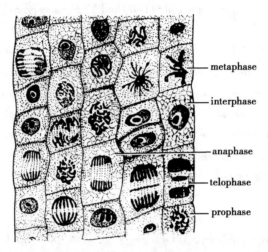

metaphase

interphase

anaphase

telophase

prophase

Fig.24-2　Mitosis of onion root tip cell

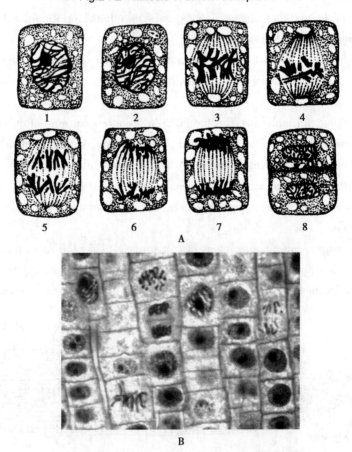

1　2　3　4

5　6　7　8

A

B

Fig.24-3　The prophase, metaphase, anaphase, telophase of mitosis of onion root tip cell

A. Pattern diagram; B. Microstructure diagram.

1.1.2.1　Interphase: Interphase cells are smaller with a clear nucleus and a more homogeneous chromatin distribution, with 1-2 nucleoli in the nucleus.

1.1.2.2　Prophase: The nucleus is enlarged, and the chromatin is filamentous and convoluted into a network. At the end of the prophase, the chromatin gradually spirals into thin thread-like chromosomes scattered in the cytoplasm; the nucleolus and nuclear envelope disappeared, and the spindle fiber appeared. Each linear chromosome is composed of two chromatids.

1.1.2.3　Metaphase: The cell begins to elongate, and all chromosomes move to the center of the cell to form the equatorial plate; the metaphase chromosome are the thickest and have the clearest structure. At this time, the spindle fiber from the two poles are connected to the centromere of the chromosome to form a spindle (not easy to see under optical microscope).

1.1.2.4　Anaphase: The cell stretches more extended, and the two chromatids split longitudinally at the centromere and separate from each other. Due to the traction of the spindle fiber, the separated two chromatids move toward the two poles. At this stage, the chromosomes are mostly V-shaped, and the tip of the V-shaped is the centromere.

1.1.2.5　Telophase: The chromatids that move to the two poles turned into chromatin, at the same time, the spindle disappears, the nuclear envelope and nucleolus reappear, and two nuclei are formed inside the cell. In the center of the cell between the two new nuclei, the Golgi body small vesicles fuse to form a cell plate, then form a cell wall separating the cytoplasm, and finally forms two daughter cells.

1.2　Animal cells: Take a transverse section slide of the uterus of equine roundworm and observe it with low power objective. It can be seen that there are many round or oval fertilized egg cells in the uterine cavity at different stages of development. Each fertilized egg cell is surrounded by a thick and pale eggshell, taking care not to mistake the eggshell for the plasma membrane. The fertilized egg cell divides in the eggshell, and there is a sizeable perivitelline space between the fertilized egg cell and the eggshell. There are polar body attachments on the surface of some fertilized egg cells or on the inner surface of the eggshell. Select fertilized egg cells in different stages of mitosis and carefully observe the structural characteristics of cells in each stage of mitosis at high power objective (Fig.24-4).

1.2.1　Interphase: There are two near round nuclei within the cytoplasm, one female pronucleus, and the other male pronucleus. The morphology of the two pronuclei is similar and difficult to distinguish. The chromatin distribution in the nucleus is relatively uniform, the nuclear envelope and nucleoli are clear, and centrioles are visible near the nucleus.

1.2.2　Prophase: Nuclear swelled. The replicated pair of centrosomes are separated from each other and move toward the cell poles. There are radiating astral ray around the centrioles (the astral microtubules on the electron microscope). The nucleolus and nuclear envelope disappear as the chromatin in the nucleus gradually condenses to form chromosomes. On the section specimens, the chromosomes are in the form of filaments, dots, or short rods, scattered randomly in the cytoplasm; sometimes, only one centrosome or no centrosome is seen due to different sections.

1.2.3　Metaphase: When the two centrosomes move toward the poles, the spindle forms and the chromosome is located in the center of the spindle. On sectioned specimens at the polar view,

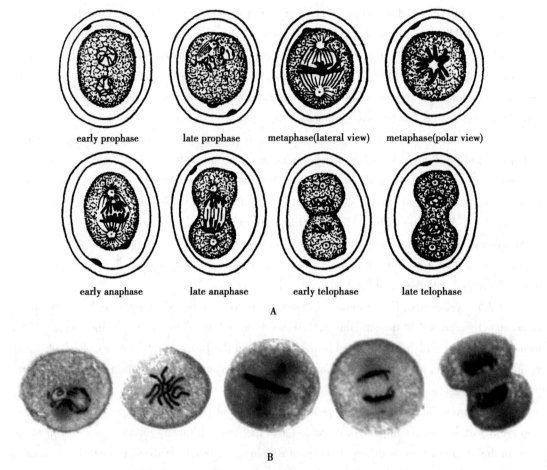

Fig.24-4　Equine roundworm fertilized egg cells mitotic process

A. Pattern diagram；B. Microstructure diagram.

chromosomes (6 in total) were radially arranged like chrysanthemums. There is a centrosome at each pole from the lateral view, and the chromosomes are arranged in a horizontal line. With fine focusing, it can be seen that the spindle fibers are connected to the centromeres on the chromosome.

1.2.4　Anaphase：After chromatid are separated from the centromere, the two sets of daughter chromosomes with the same number move toward the cell poles under spindle fibers traction. Microscopically, the chromatids are oriented with their centromeres toward one pole and their two arms toward the middle of the cell, forming a V shape. The two sets of daughter chromosomes, like two opposing combs, move to the poles. At the end of anaphase, the plasma membrane in the middle of the cell invaginate.

1.2.5　Telophase：The chromatids that reached the poles unwind into chromatin, the spindle and astral ray disappear, the nucleolus and nuclear envelope reappear, and the constriction of the plasma membrane deepens, and finally the cell constricts to form 2 daughter cells.

2. Meiosis　Observing of specimens of male locust sperm nest：The male locust sperm nest is comprised multiple cylindrical seminiferous tubules, and locust spermatogenesis occurs from the

epithelium of seminiferous tubule. There are two ends of the tubule seminiferous:blind end is free, and the other end(attachment end) is opens to the vas deferens. On a well-made tabletting, starting from the free blind end, you can see spermatogonium, spermatocyte, spermatid, and sperm in sequence. First, distinguish the different locations of the tubule seminiferous at low power objective, and then switch to high power objective or oil immersion objective, to identify the cell types and the periods to which they belong, based on their structure.

2.1　Spermatogonium:Spermatogonium proliferate through mitosis and are located at the free end of the tubule seminiferous with small, round or oval somata, and large, deep staining nucleus and irregular arrangement of chromatin in lumps. Every spermatogonium contains the same number of chromosomes as somatic cell.

2.2　Primary spermatocyte:Primary spermatocytes develop from spermatogonium that undergo anagen differentiation, and have the same number of chromosomes as spermatogonia. Each primary spermatocyte form two secondary spermatocytes by meiosis Ⅰ. Similar to the mitotic process, meiosis Ⅰ can also be divided into four stages:prophase, metaphase, anaphase, and telophase. The difference from mitosis is that prophase Ⅰ is long, complex with nuclear changes, the most characteristic stage of meiosis

2.2.1　Prophase Ⅰ:According to the morphological changes of chromosomes in the nucleus, prophase Ⅰ can be divided into the following subphase:

2.2.1.1　Leptotene:The chromatin is condensed into elongated linear chromosomes, and they are wrapped into a cluster, so the nucleus is large and light in color, and difficult to distinguish. On the filamentous chromosomes, beaded chromomere can be seen. Nucleolus can also be seen in the nucleus (Fig.24-5). The microscopic characteristics of specimens in this stage are as follows: chromosomes are filamentous or villi with light color.

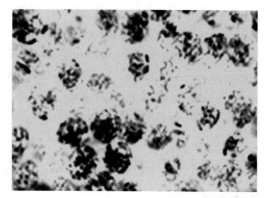

Fig.24-5　Leptotene

2.2.1.2　Zygotene:In this stage, the nucleus is larger, and the chromosomes morphology is not much changed from the leptotene, and they are still fine and long;each pair of homologous chromosomes begins to pair from one end, and the paired-end gathers on one side of the nucleus, the other end spreads out to form a flower bundle like shape. The result of the pairing is the formation of 11 tetrads, which are also called bivalent. The X chromosome condenses into an X body which is present at the inner edge of the nuclear envelope, due to an inability to pair. Due to the short duration of this stage, it is usually difficult to observe. The microscopic features of specimens at this stage are as follows:Chromosomes are thin and long, and Some segments of two homologous chromosomes are sometimes clearly seen side by side (Fig.24-6).

2.2.1.3　Pachytene:The paired homologous chromosomes (tetrad) shorten and thicken, and the chromosomes in the entire nucleus appear sparse (Fig.24-7). Crossover is seen because of

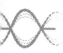

the exchange that can occur between non-sister chromatids at this stage. The microscopic features of specimens at this stage are as follows: the chromosomes as thick lines, and chromomere are often seen.

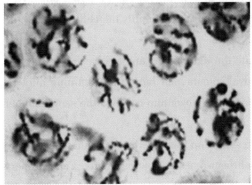

Fig.24-6 Zygotene

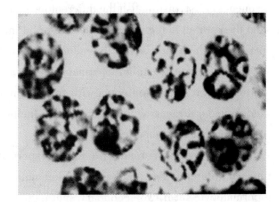

Fig.24-7 Pachytene

2.2.1.4 Diplotene: The chromosomes became thicker and shorter, and the surface was not smooth, like villiform. Eleven tetrads and one X chromosome can be distinguished. The two homologous chromosomes of the tetrad are tightly linked, and it is difficult to distinguish them. During this stage, homologous chromosomes began to separate, but the separation was incomplete due to the chiasma between non-sister chromatids of homologous chromosomes. Chiasma is the performance of local exchange between non-sister chromatids. As the chiasma gradually extends toward the end, one or two points on the chromosome cross together in various shapes such as X, O, or $\propto$ (Fig.24-8). The X chromosome is rod-shaped and has no chiasma. The microscopic features of specimens at this stage are as follows: the chromosomes are more condensed and stubby than those in pachytene, larger loops, octagons, rods and other morphologies are seen, and the loops of ring chromosomes are large and thin.

2.2.1.5 Diakinesis: Chromosomes are condensed and stubby, surface smooth, morphologically diverse, and mostly distributed around the nucleus. The tetrads are clear and countable. The chiasma is further extended toward both ends to form special images such as O, V, X, and Y. The nucleolus and nuclear envelope disappeared (Fig.24-9).

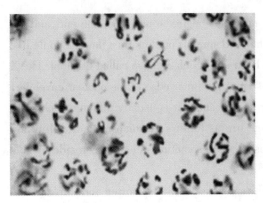

Fig.24-8 Diplotene

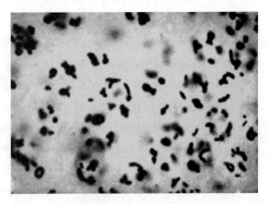

Fig.24-9 Diakinesis

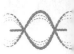

2.2.2　Metaphase Ⅰ：The tetrads are highly condensed, with smooth edges, arranged in the center of the cell, plate-like on lateral view, and hollow flower-like on polar view. The nuclear envelope completely disappeared, the spindle appeared, and the centromere was connected with the spindle fibers(Fig.24-10).

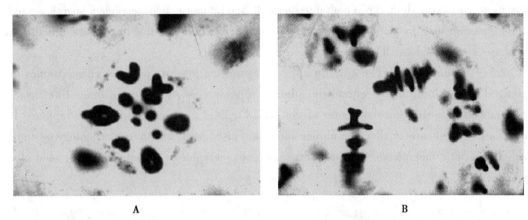

A   B

Fig.24-10　Meiosis metaphase Ⅰ

A. Pattern diagram；B. Microstructure diagram.

2.2.3　Anaphase Ⅰ：The two homologous chromosomes of the tetrads are separated, and the non-homologous chromosomes are randomly combined into two groups, with 11 chromosomes in one group and 12 chromosomes in the other. Pulled by the spindle fibers, the two sets of chromosomes move toward the poles, respectively(Fig.24-11). On Polar view, the chromosomes are arranged in a chrysanthemum shape at two poles. The microscopic features of specimens at this stage are as follows：two sets of V-shaped chromosomes can be seen.

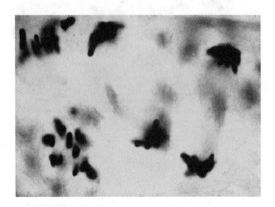

Fig.24-11　Meiosis anaphase Ⅰ

2.2.4　Telophase Ⅰ：The chromosomes that reach the poles are untwisted into chromatin, the nucleolus and nuclear envelope are formed again. The cell was elongated and the middle part of the cell shrinks so that the cytoplasm is divided equally to form two smaller diad, namely secondary spermatocyte.

2.3　Secondary spermatocyte：After completion of the meiosis Ⅰ, the two secondary spermatocytes are formed and contain 11 and 12 chromosomes, respectively, that is, the number of chromosome has been halved(n=11+X, or n=11+0).

2.3.1　Interphase Ⅱ：The secondary spermatocytes generated by meiosis Ⅰ are in the interphase, and the interphase is very short, without DNA replication, directly enter meiosis Ⅱ. Meiosis Ⅱ is also divided into four phases：prophase, metaphase, anaphase and telophase, and its morphological changes are similar to those of somatic mitosis. However, in terms of

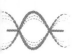

cell morphology, the number of chromosomes is reduced by half, and the cell is significantly smaller.

2.3.2　Prophase Ⅱ: Chromosomes show a tendency to separate, arranged like petals, so that the cells of prophase Ⅱ appear solid flower-like. The nucleolus and nuclear envelope disappeared. This stage is also very short. Since both interphase Ⅱ and prophase Ⅱ of secondary spermatocyte in male locusts are short-lived, they are not easily observed; it is even possible to progress directly from telophase Ⅰ to metaphase Ⅱ.

2.3.3　Metaphase Ⅱ: The spindle appears again. On lateral view, the chromosomes are arranged in a column at the equatorial plane; on polar view, the chromosomes like flowers are arranged in a circle in the center of the cell (Fig.24-12). Compared with metaphase Ⅰ, metaphase Ⅱ cells are smaller; the chromosomes are also small, and their morphology is similar to that of mitotic metaphase. On the microscope, two metaphase Ⅱ cells are often seen close together.

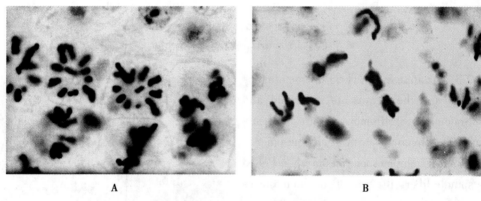

A   B

Fig.24-12　Meiosis metaphase Ⅱ

A. Polar view; B. Lateral view.

2.3.4　Anaphase Ⅱ: Due to the traction of the spindle fibers, the two group daughter chromosomes (chromatids) formed by the centromeric split of each chromosome move to the poles of the cell respectively. Each group has n (n=11 or 12) daughter chromosomes, the number of which is half of that of primary spermatocytes (23) (Fig.24-13). The microscopic features of specimens at this stage are as follows: two sets of rod-shaped daughter chromosomes can be seen.

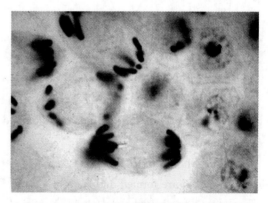

Fig.24-13　Meiosis anaphase Ⅱ

2.3.5　Telophase Ⅱ: The two sets of daughter chromosomes that move to the poles unwind and coalesce into clusters to form chromatin, the nuclear envelope and the nucleolus reappear to form a new nucleus, in turn forms 2 round spermatids. Microscopically, spermatids with larger nuclei are smaller than secondary spermatocytes

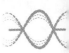

（Fig.24-14）. Four immediately adjacent spermatids, i.e. 4 spermatids formed from 1 primary spermatocyte undergoing meiosis Ⅰ and meiosis Ⅱ, were sometimes seen, 2 of which contained 11 daughter chromosomes and the other 2 contained 12 daughter chromosomes. Four daughter cells formed by meiosis are also called tetrad. To this point, meiosis Ⅱ is completed.

2.4　Sperm: The spermatids initially changed from round to round headed long tailed, then gradually changed to oval headed long tailed, finally formed spermatozoa of elongated spindle shaped heads and long tails（Fig.24-15）.

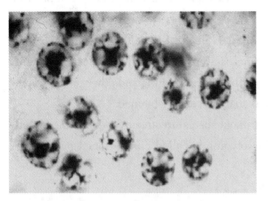

Fig.24-14　Morphology of spermatids

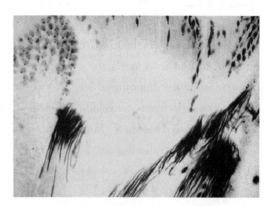

Fig.24-15　Morphology of sperm

【Analysis and thinking】

1. Compare the number of chromosomes, chromatids, and DNA molecules in primary spermatocytes, secondary spermatocytes, and sperm cells.

2. Compare the similarities and differences between meiosis and mitosis.

【Experimental report】

1. Draw a cell structure diagram for the interphase, prophase, metaphase（polar view, lateral view）, anaphase, and telophase of mitosis separately.

2. Draw a cell structure diagram for metaphase Ⅰ, metaphase Ⅱ, and diplotene and diakinesis of prophase Ⅰ in spermatocytes meiosis of male locusts separately.

Experiment 25　Karyotyping of Human Non-banding Chromosome

【Purpose and requirements】

1. Be familiar with the principles of human peripheral blood lymphocyte culture and preparation of chromosome samples.

2. Be familiar with non-banding chromosome karyotypic features and methods of karyotyping analysis methods of normal people.

【Experimental principle】

Among the cellular components of human peripheral blood, only white blood cells are nucleated whereas in leukocytes, only lymphocytes（mainly small lymphocytes）have the potential to divide.

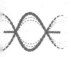

When the cell enters the division phase, the chromatin in the interphase's nucleus is gradually folded and compressed to form chromosomes. In the metaphase of mitosis, the chromosomes show typically short and thick structure.

The addition of the mitogenic stimulant Phytohemagglutinin (PHA) to the culture medium of peripheral blood lymphocytes can transform the lymphocytes that have the potential to divide and are in the G_0 phase into lymphoblasts with the ability to divide; and then the lymphoblasts enter the cell cycle. When the cell culture process enters the logarithmic growth phase, adding the spindle inhibitor colchicine to the culture medium can arrests the lymphocytes in the metaphase of mitosis.

When harvesting the cells, the cells are treated with 0.075mol/L KCl solution, whose hypotonic effect make the cells swell, the cytoplasmic membrane easily rupture, and chromosomes evenly disperse while the dropping tablet. After centrifugation, fixation, sectioning and other processes, the chromosome specimens convenient for observation and analysis can be obtained.

The prepared pieces of chromosome specimens, without special treatment, and staining directly followed by recognition under a microscope and karyotyping is called chromosomal non-banded karyotyping.

【 Experimental supplies 】

1. Materials and reagents　Video data for the method of human chromosome specimen preparation, non-banding chromosome specimen slide, non-banding chromosome karyotype photographs.

2. Equipments　Microscope, cedar oil (or liquid paraffin), absolute ethanol (or ether-ethanol mixture), lens paper, waste liquid tank, scissors, tweezers, glue, toothpicks.

【 Experimental procedures 】

1. Watching the video data for the method of human chromosome specimen preparation.

2. Observing non-banding chromosome specimen slide　A non-banding chromosome specimen slide is first viewed at low power objective, then select metaphase that chromosomes are well morphology, uniform dispersion and without cytosolic background to carefully observe by oil immersion objective. According to the chromosome image seen on the microscope, draw a quick line drawing of the chromosome distribution on the experimental report paper (Fig.25-1). The position, relative length, and centromere position of each chromosome in the figure should be as closely as possible to that observed microscopically.

2.1　Chromosome count: Count the chromosomes based on the quick line drawing to determine whether there is abnormality in chromosome number. The number of chromosomes in normal human somatic cells is 2n=46, in which there is 22 pairs of autosomes and 1 pair of sex chromosomes. The karyotype expression is 46,XY, for normal male and 46,XX for normal female.

2.2　Chromosome morphological structure analysis: Each chromosome contains two chromatids, which are connected through centromere. The chromosome structure extending from the centromere to chromosomal end is called chromosome arm. The chromosome arm includes a short arm (indicated by p) and a long arm (indicated by q).

According to the centromeric location, human chromosomes are divided into 3 categories:

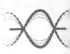

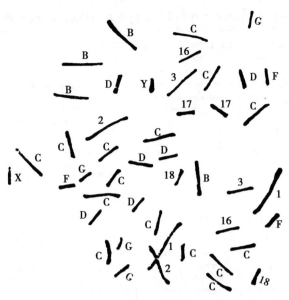

Fig.25-1 Quick line drawing of chromosome distribution

the metacentric chromosome, whose long arm is almost equal to the short arm; the submetacentric chromosome, whose long arm can be clearly distinguished from the short arm; the acrocentric chromosome, whose short arm is extremely short, centromere is almost at the tip of the chromosome, and sometimes the satellite can be seen on the short arm.

On oil immersion objective, observe the morphological structure and the location of secondary constriction of chromosome, and the presence or absence of chromosomal structural aberrations such as break, deletion, duplication, translocation, inversion, ring chromosome and isochromosome. According to the morphological and structural features of non-banding chromosomes, mark chromosome number or group number next to the chromosome in the quick line drawing. When observing non-banded chromosomes, the chromosomes that can be accurately distinguished include chromosome 1, 2, 3, 16, 17, 18, and Y.

3. Analysis of non-banding chromosome karyotype photographs by cutting and pasting   To determine whether the examined individual has chromosomal number or structural abnormality, the best mitotic metaphase cell is often microscopically sought, photomicrographed, and enlarged photographs; each chromosome on the photograph is cropped, and the chromosomes were pasted to their corresponding positions on the karyotyping table according to the rules of An International System for Human Cytogenetic Nomenclature (ISCN) and characteristics such as chromosome size and centromere position. This procedure is called karyotype photograph clipping and pasting analysis, short form karyotyping. ISCN divides human chromosomes into seven groups (A, B, C, D, E, F, G), the chromosomes in each group and the structural characteristics of chromosomes are shown in Table 25-1.

Table 25-1　Human non-banding chromosome structure characteristics

Group	NO.	Size	Centromere Type	Satellite	Supplement
A	1,3	maximum	metacentric	×	No.3 is slightly smaller than No.1
	2		submetacentric		
B	4,5	second largest	submetacentric	×	short arm of group B is shorter than that of group C
C	6-12,X	medium	submetacentric	×	No.9,10 and 12 have shorter arm The size of X is between NO.7 and 8
D	13-15	medium	acrocentric	√	They are similar in length and difficult to distinguish
E	16	small	metacentric	×	No.18 has shorter arm than No.17
	17,18		submetacentric		
F	19,20	second smallest	metacentric	×	Hard to distinguish
G	21,22	minimum	acrocentric	√	The two long arms are often bifurcated. They are difficult to distinguish
	Y			×	The two long arms are often close together

　　Karyotype analysis is carried out according to the order of counting the total number of chromosomes, judging gender, and cutting and pasting karyotype photographs. If the number of chromosome is normal with no obvious structural abnormality, it can be considered a normal karyotype. According to the characteristics of the G group chromosomes, if there is 5 (No.21 × 2, No.22 × 2, and 1 Y chromosome) of the smallest acrocentric chromosome (G group), it can be judged as a male karyotype; if there is 4 of the G group, it is female karyotype.

　　Before cutting and pasting non-banding chromosome karyotype photographs, first find groups A, B, D, E, F and G in turn according to chromosomes' structural characteristics in each group, and the remaining chromosomes are determined as group C; and then the group number is marked next to each chromosome with a pencil, each chromosome is sheared along with the chromosome's group number with scissors, each group of chromosomes was arranged in order of size; if found to be arranged with errors, adjustments are possible; finally, clip the chromosome's group number, arrange each chromosome in the chromosome karyotyping table's corresponding position, in glue. Pasting the chromosome should hold the short arm up, the long arm down, and the centromere in a straight line (Fig.25-2, Fig.25-3). The shearing process should be attentive, preventing the loss of chromosomes.

　　4. Chromosome measurement　Measure the length of the short and long arm of each chromosome on the karyotyping table with a ruler, then calculate the relative length, arm ratio, and centromere index of each chromosome.

　　(1) Arm ratio = long arm length/short arm length.

　　(2) Centromere index = (short arm length/full length of the chromosome) × 100%.

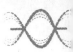

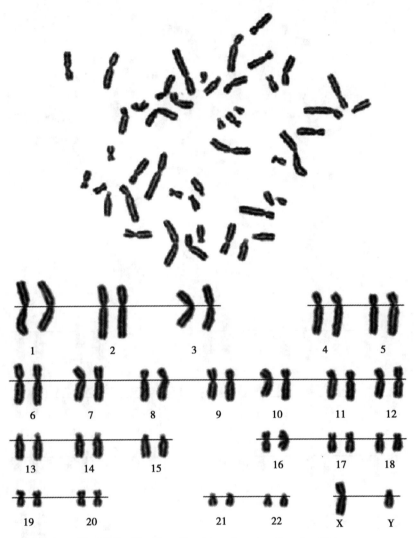

Fig.25-2   Non-banding karyotype in normal males

（3）Relative length=〔length of each chromosome/total chromosome length in haploid cell（22+X）〕× 100%.

【Analysis and thinking】

1. What are the roles of PHA and colchicine each in the process of lymphocyte culture?

2. What is the effect of treating cells with 0.075mol/L KCl solution when harvesting cells?

【Experimental report】

1. Draw a quick line drawing of non-banding chromosomes on the microscope（mark the number or group number next to the chromosomes）.

2. Karyotype analysis：Cut and paste the photographs of non-banding chromosome of a normal females for karyotype analysis（Fig.25-4，Fig.8-5 at the end of the book）.

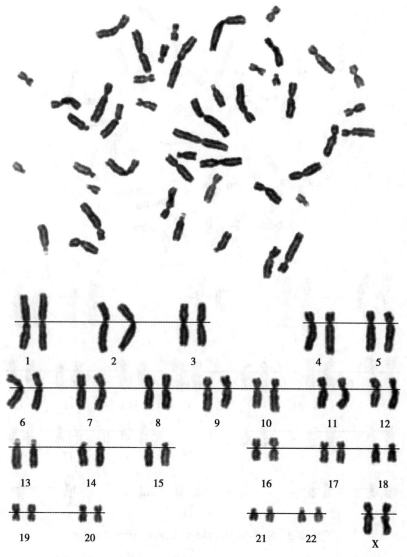

Fig.25-3　Non-banding karyotype in normal females

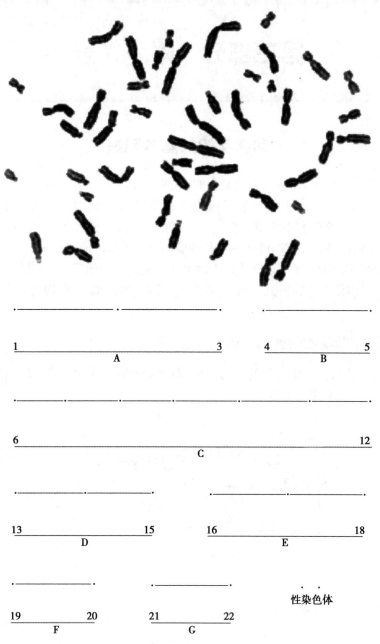

Fig.25-4 Karyotyping of non-banding chromosome in normal females by cutting and pasting photographs

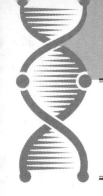

第三部分　附　　录

动物实验的基本知识

医学科学研究包括临床研究和实验研究,这两种途径均离不开动物实验。动物实验方法的采用和发展促进了医学科学的发展,解决了许多以往不能解决的实际问题。比如,由于在肿瘤的移植、免疫等研究中使用了裸鼠、悉生动物和无菌动物,从而在各种恶性肿瘤的病因,尤其是化学致癌、病毒致癌、肿瘤免疫和肿瘤治疗等方面的研究取得了令人瞩目的进展。在医学研究中采用动物模型可以使很多人体上非常复杂的问题简单化;临床上少见的疾病,应用动物实验可以随时进行研究。因此,作为一个医学生,应掌握动物实验的基本知识和基本操作技能。

一、描述实验动物的解剖术语

为了描述实验动物机体内部的不同结构,通常依据动物体的长度、宽度和厚度,在动物身体上做出相互垂直的切面(附图-1A)。

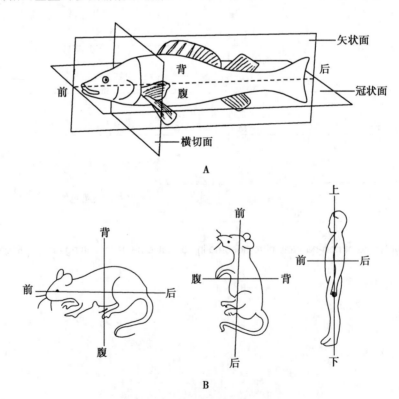

附图 -1　实验动物的切面与方位

A. 实验动物的切面;B. 解剖方位。

（一）矢状面

矢状面是沿着动物的头部至尾部的切面,该切面将动物分为左右两部分。当实验动物腹面向上时,实验动物的左右与面对动物的实验者的左右相反。如果切面在动物体的正中线通过就称为正中面,它把动物体分成左右对称的两部分。机体的任何部分,近正中者称内侧,远中者称外侧。

（二）冠状面

冠状面也是沿着动物的头部至尾部切面,但与矢状面垂直。冠状面将动物体分成背侧和腹侧两部分。

（三）横切面

横切面与矢状面、冠状面垂直,将动物体分为前后两部分。体内器官朝向头部的一端称前端(头端),朝向尾部的一端称后端(尾端)。

另外,为了说明体内器官所在部位距离体表的远近,将近皮肤者称浅层;反之,称深层。某一系统的主要部分称中枢,由主要部分延伸出的结构部分称外周。比如,神经系统的脑和脊髓称中枢,周围神经称外周;循环系统的心脏为中枢,血管为外周。

值得注意的是,上述各种术语是针对动物的,与人体解剖学的描述术语不完全相同,如人的头端为上不为前,足端为下不为后(见附图 -1B)。

二、动物实验的基本操作

（一）实验动物的抓取与固定

正确地抓取并固定动物,是为了不损害动物,不影响观察指标,并防止被动物咬伤,保证实验顺利进行。抓取和固定动物的方法依实验内容和动物种类而定。抓取固定动物前,必须对各种动物的一般习性有所了解,抓取、固定时既要小心、仔细,又要大胆、敏捷。以下简介蛙类、家兔和小鼠的抓取与固定方法。

1. 蛙类　抓取蛙时,宜用左手将动物背部贴紧手掌固定,以中指、环指、小指压住其左腹侧和后肢,拇指和示指分别压住左、右前肢(附图 -2),右手进行操作。

抓取蟾蜍时,应注意勿挤压其两侧耳部的毒腺,以免毒液射入眼中。实验时,如需长时间观察,可破坏其脊髓,或麻醉后用大头针固定在蛙板上或蜡盘中。依实验需要采取俯卧位或仰卧位固定。

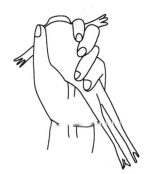

附图 -2　蛙的抓取方法

2. 家兔　实验家兔一般饲养在笼内,所以抓取比较方便。一般以右手抓住兔颈部的毛皮提起,然后左手托其臀部或腹部,让其体重的大部分重量集中到左手上(附图 -3)。不正确的抓取方法将造成家兔损伤。

家兔的固定分为盒式、台式和马蹄式 3 种。盒式固定适用于兔耳采血、耳血管注射等。若进行血压测量、呼吸等实验或手术,则需台式固定:将兔固定在兔台上,拉直四肢,用粗棉绳活结将其绑在兔台四周的固定木块上;头以固定夹固定或用一根粗棉绳挑过门齿绑在兔台铁柱上。马蹄形固定多用于腰背部,尤其是颅脑部的实验,固定时先剪去两侧眼眶下部的毛皮,暴露颧骨突起,调节固定器两端钉形金属棒,使其正好嵌在突起下方的凹陷处;然后在适当的高度固定金属棒。马蹄形固定器可使兔取背卧位或腹卧位,是实验中较常采用的固定方式。在进行家兔解剖实验时,常将家兔处死后仰卧固定在解剖盘中。

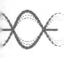

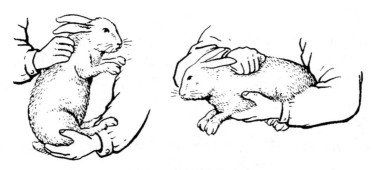

附图 -3 家兔的抓取方法

3. 小鼠 小鼠温顺,一般不会咬人,抓取时先用右手抓取鼠尾提起,置于鼠笼或实验台上向后拉,在其向前爬行时,用左手拇指和示指抓住小鼠的两耳和颈部皮肤(附图 -4A),将鼠体置于左手手心中,把后肢拉直,环指按住鼠尾,小指按住后腿即可。有经验者可直接用左手钩起鼠尾,迅速以拇指、示指和中指捏住其耳后颈背部皮肤(附图 -4B)。这种手中固定方式,能进行灌胃、皮下注射、肌内注射和腹腔注射以及其他实验操作。

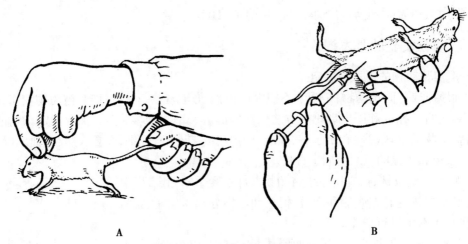

A   B

附图 -4 小鼠的抓取与腹腔注射
A. 抓取方法;B. 腹腔注射方法。

进行解剖、手术、心脏采血和尾静脉注射时,则需将小鼠做一定形式的固定。解剖、手术或心脏采血时,可使小鼠取背卧位(必要时先行麻醉),用大头针将鼠前后肢依次固定在蜡板上。尾静脉注射时,可用固定架固定。根据小鼠大小选择合适的固定架;打开筒盖,手提鼠尾,让鼠头对准鼠筒口送入筒内;调节鼠筒长短,使尾巴露出,固定好筒盖,这样即可进行尾静脉注射或采血等操作(附图 -5)。

(二)实验动物的给药途径
根据实验目的、实验动物的类型和药物剂型的不同,可采用不同的给药途径。现简介如下几种:
1. 皮下注射 注射时用左手拇指和示指提起皮肤,将注射器的针头刺入皮下,注入药液。根据不同动物,可在不同部位进针:狗、猫多在大腿外侧,大白鼠可在侧下腹部,兔在背部或耳根部。

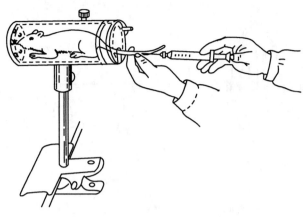

附图 -5 小鼠固定架固定与尾静脉注射

2. 皮内注射 皮内注射时需将注射的局部脱去被毛、消毒,然后用左手拇指和示指按住皮肤并使之绷紧,在两指之间,用结核菌素注射器连 4.5 号细针头,紧贴皮肤表层刺入皮内,然后再向上挑起并再稍刺入,即可注射药液,此时可见皮肤表面鼓起一白色小皮丘。

3. 肌内注射 肌内注射应选肌肉发达、无大血管通过的部位,一般多选臀部。注射时,垂直、迅速刺入肌肉,回抽针栓如无回血,即可进行注射。给小白鼠、大白鼠等小动物作肌内注射时,用左手抓住鼠两耳和头部皮肤,右手取连有针头的注射器,将针头刺入大腿外侧肌肉,将药液注入。

4. 腹腔注射 对大白鼠、小白鼠进行腹腔注射时,以左手抓住动物,使腹部向上,右手将注射针头于左(或右)后腹部刺入皮下,使针头向前推 0.5~1.0cm,再以 45° 角穿过腹肌,缓缓注入药液(见附图 -4B)。为避免伤及内脏,可使动物处于头低位,使内脏移向前腹。若对家兔行腹腔注射,进针部位应在后腹部的腹中线外侧 1cm 处。

5. 静脉注射

(1)蛙或蟾蜍:将蛙或蟾蜍脑脊髓破坏后,仰卧固定于蛙板或蜡盘上,沿腹中线稍左剪开腹肌,可见到腹静脉贴着腹壁肌肉后行,将注射针头沿血管平行方向刺入即可(附图 -6)。

(2)兔:兔耳部血管分布清晰,耳中央有粗大的动脉,耳边缘为静脉(附图 -7A)。内缘静脉深,不好固定,故不用;外缘静脉表浅易固定,常用。先拔去注射部位的被毛,用手指轻弹兔耳,使静脉充盈;也可用蘸水的湿纱布或乙醇(酒精)棉球擦拭外缘静脉处皮肤,使静脉充盈。左手示指和中指夹住静脉的近端,拇指和环指夹住静脉的远端,右手持注射器从静脉的远端刺入(附图 -7B),移动拇指于针头上以固定针头,放开示指和中指,将药物注入,然后拔出针头,用手压迫针眼片刻。如一次注射失败,

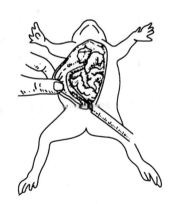

附图 -6 蛙腹壁静脉注射

可在原注射处的近心方向再注射。空气栓塞法处死家兔的基本操作与此相似。

(3)小鼠和大鼠:一般采用尾静脉注射。鼠尾静脉有 3 根,左侧、右侧和背侧各 1 根,左右两侧尾静脉比较容易固定,多采用;背侧一根也可采用,但位置不容易固定。操作时先将动物固定在鼠筒内,使尾巴露出;尾用 45~50℃的温水浸泡 30s 或用乙醇(酒精)擦拭使血管扩张及表皮角质软化,以左手拇指和示指捏住鼠尾两侧使静脉充盈,用中指从下面托起

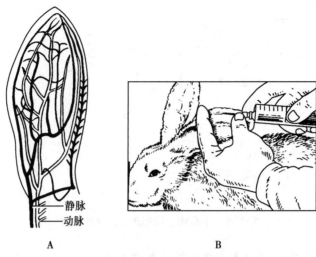

附图 -7 家兔的耳部血管分布及耳缘静脉注射方法

A. 耳部血管分布；B. 耳缘静脉注射方法。

尾巴，环指和小指夹住尾巴的末梢，右手持 4.5 号细针头的注射器，使针头与静脉平行（小于 30° 角），从尾下 1/4 处（距尾尖 2~3cm）进针（见附图 -5）。此处皮薄易于刺入，先缓缓注入少量药液，如无阻力，表明针头已进入静脉，可继续注入。注射完毕后把尾部向注射侧弯曲以止血。如需反复注射，应尽可能从末端开始，以后向尾根部方向移动注射。

（三）实验动物的麻醉

在动物实验前，需对动物进行麻醉。由于动物种属间存在差异，故所采用的麻醉方法和选用的麻醉剂亦有不同。

1. 吸入全麻法 用 1 块圆玻璃板和 1 个钟罩或 1 个有盖密闭的标本瓶作为挥发性麻醉剂的容器，麻醉剂多选用乙醚。在上述容器内放置数个干棉球，将乙醚倒在其中，然后把待麻醉动物投入，4~6min 即可麻醉。麻醉后应立即取出，并准备一个盛有乙醚棉球的小烧杯，在动物麻醉变浅时，套在动物鼻子上使其补吸麻醉剂。本法最适用于大、小鼠的短期麻醉，以及青蛙、蟾蜍的麻醉。

2. 注射全麻法 非挥发性麻醉剂如苯巴比妥钠、戊巴比妥钠、氨基甲酸乙酯、水合氯醛，以及中药麻醉剂如洋金花等，可用做腹腔和静脉注射麻醉。注射法操作简便，是实验室常用的方法之一。腹腔注射多用于大鼠、小鼠和豚鼠，较大的动物，如兔、狗等则多用静脉注射麻醉。

3. 局部麻醉法 猫的局部麻醉一般应用 0.5%~1% 盐酸普鲁卡因注射，黏膜表面麻醉宜用 2% 盐酸可卡因。兔的眼球手术时，可于结膜囊滴入 0.02% 盐酸可卡因，数秒即可出现麻醉。狗的麻醉用 0.5%~1.0% 盐酸普鲁卡因注射，眼、鼻、咽喉表面麻醉可用 2% 盐酸可卡因。

（四）实验动物的处死

1. 蛙类 蛙类处死常采用捣毁脊髓法。操作时，左手用湿布将蛙包住，露出头部，用示指按其头部前端，拇指按压背部，使头前俯；右手持金属探针自头前端沿中线向尾端依次刺触，触及凹陷处即为枕骨大孔所在。将探针由枕骨大孔垂直刺入，刺破皮肤即达枕骨大孔。将探针尖端转向头侧，向前探入颅腔，然后向各方搅动，以捣毁脑组织。如探针确在颅腔内，实验者会感到探针在四面皆壁的腔内。脑组织捣毁后，将探针退出，再由枕骨大孔刺入，并转向尾侧,与脊柱平行刺入椎管,破坏脊髓。脑和脊髓是否完全破坏,可根据四肢肌肉的紧张性是否完全消失来判断。拔出探针后,用一小干棉球将针孔堵住,防止出血。

操作过程中要防止毒腺分泌物射入操作者眼中,如不慎射入,应立即用生理盐水冲洗。

2. 大鼠和小鼠

（1）颈椎脱臼法:操作者左手拇指和示指用力向下按住鼠头,右手抓住鼠尾根部用力向后拉,使颈椎脱位、脊髓拉断,鼠便立即死亡。

（2）断头法:操作者戴棉纱手套,右手握住鼠头部,左手握住背部,露出颈部,助手用剪刀在鼠颈部将鼠头剪断。

（3）击打法:右手抓住鼠尾,提起,用力摔击其头部,鼠痉挛后立即死亡。用小木槌用力击打鼠头部也可致死。

（4）化学致死法:0.2%~0.5% 一氧化碳吸入,或每只静脉注射 25% 氯化钾溶液 0.6ml 均可致死。吸入乙醚、氯仿也可致死。

3. 兔、猫、狗

（1）空气栓塞法:静脉内注入一定量的空气,动物可因血管内空气栓塞而死亡。空气经静脉回流到心脏,随着心脏的跳动,空气与血液相混合,血液形成泡沫状,经血液循环流到全身;随着动脉的分支变细,空气栓塞阻塞动脉的分支,导致严重的血液循环障碍,动物很快死亡。一般兔静脉注射 5ml 空气,猫静脉注射 20~40ml 空气即可死亡,狗静脉注射 80~100ml 空气可致死亡。

（2）化学致死法:静脉注射一定量的氯化钾溶液,可使动物心肌失去收缩能力,心脏急性扩张,致心脏停搏而死亡。常用氯化钾溶液浓度为 10%。成年兔静脉注射 20ml 可致死,成年狗静脉注射 20~30ml 可致死。静脉注射一定量的甲醛溶液,可使动物血液内蛋白凝固,全身血液循环障碍,严重缺氧而死亡。成年狗注入 10% 的甲醛 20ml 即可死亡。

三、常用动物解剖器械及其使用

（一）解剖刀

解剖刀用作各种切割、剥离与剔除软组织等,解剖刀由刀片和刀柄两部分构成。使用时,以拇指和示指、中指相对握持,如握笔姿势(附图 -8A)。使用解剖刀进行解剖时,必须注意刀刃方向和插入深度,避免伤及需要保留的组织;在剥离皮肤时,应使刀刃朝皮肤方向,这样可避免损伤皮下的肌肉和血管。

（二）解剖剪

解剖剪用作各种切口及中空性器官的剪断等。使用时,拇指和环指穿入柄部的孔环,示指紧贴剪轴的外侧,以保持剪股平稳(见附图 -8B)。在做腹壁切口时,应使剪尖上翘,以免损伤内脏及血管。

解剖刀和解剖剪一般只作解剖动物软组织用,要求经常保持锋利、清洁。

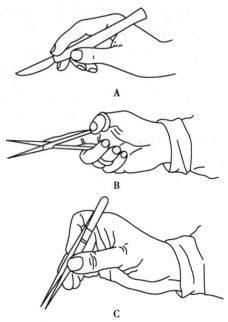

附图 -8 常用解剖器械的执法

A. 解剖刀的执法;B. 解剖剪的执法;C. 解剖镊的执法。

（三）解剖镊

解剖镊常用来夹住和提起皮肤及其他组织以利于剥离,在暴露血管和神经时,用它来剔除结缔组织。执法是拇指相对示指、中指握持镊子中部,镊尖向下(见附图 -8C)。在剔除结缔组织和脂肪组织时,应两手各执一把,用其中一把镊子夹住一部分组织,另一把细心地将要剔除的结缔组织剥离。镊子有尖头、钝头和弯头 3 种。清除血管周围的结缔组织时,要用钝头镊子,以免损伤内脏及血管。

（四）解剖针

解剖针用作各种管道的探通及拨动、剔除和剥离组织等,执法与解剖刀的执法相同。使用时,入针要浅,拨动要轻,切勿刺破血管。

（五）止血钳

止血钳也称血管钳,用于夹住不慎损伤的较大血管,以达到止血的目的,执法与解剖剪执法相同。

（六）骨剪

骨剪用作剪断骨骼或软骨。使用时,拇指和其余四指相对握持剪柄,剪刃和骨面相交。

四、动物解剖的基本要求

动物解剖前除准备好有关器械外,重要的是掌握所要解剖动物的解剖知识,了解先做什么,后做什么。也就是说,解剖前要做到心中有数。

解剖过程中,要细心和耐心,严格按实验指南介绍的方法与步骤进行。解剖动物的过程是观察认识动物器官结构的过程,除可将影响观察的脂肪和结缔组织剔除外,应尽可能保持器官结构的完整性,不能乱切乱剪器官结构。

解剖过程中,出血是难免的,但应尽量避免较大血管的出血。只要有出血,就要随时止血,否则出血部位血糊糊一片,影响观察。止血方法依出血血管的大小而定,毛细血管出血可用温热的纱布按压出血处;较大血管的出血先用血管钳钳夹,然后用细线结扎;出血较多时,先用湿纱布将血吸净,看准出血部位,再用血管钳钳夹。

辨认血管、神经是进行动物解剖的重要内容之一,因此,分离血管、神经是非常重要的。操作时,先用止血钳将血管或神经周围的结缔组织稍加分离,再在神经或血管附近的结缔组织中插入大小适合的止血钳,顺着神经或血管走行方向扩张止血钳,逐渐使其周围结缔组织剥离。这种分离方法称为钝性分离。切不可用解剖刀、解剖剪直接切割周围组织,更不能直接伤及神经或血管。

解剖完毕,应将动物尸体及残骸放到指定部位,统一处理;所用器械要认真清洗并将水迹擦干,以防锈蚀。

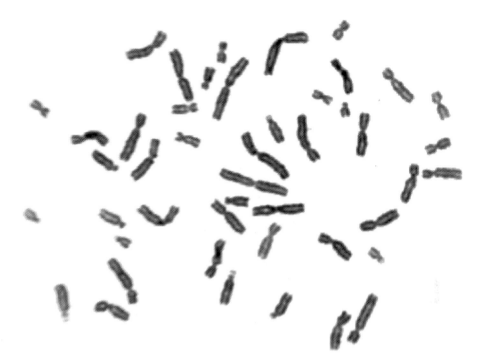

图 8-5　正常女性非显带染色体核型照片
Fig. 8-5　Non-banding karyotype in normal females

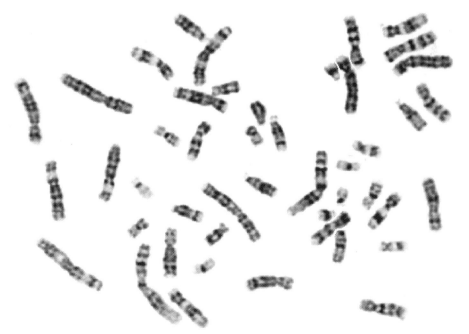

图 14-5　正常男性 G 显带染色体核型照片

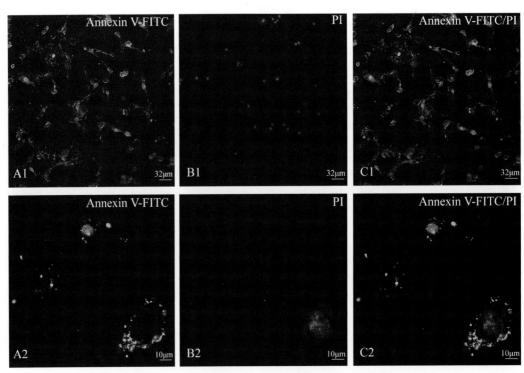

图 11-1　H₂O₂ 诱导的胶质瘤 U251 细胞凋亡（Annexin V-FITC/PI 染色）